Angina: A Systematic Guide to Investigation and Treatment

Editors
Henry Purcell
Sam Kaddoura

Mosby

LONDON • EDINBURGH • NEW YORK • PHILADELPHIA • ST LOUIS • SYDNEY • TORONTO • 2001

Preface

Angina pectoris is sometimes described as cardiac chest pain caused by transient myocardial ischaemia due to atherosclerotic (in over 90% of cases) or non-atherosclerotic coronary artery disease (e.g. coronary spasm). Such a definition belies the complexities of the disease process and the difficulties in making the correct diagnosis. The intention of this text is to provide medical students, general practitioners, hospital doctors, and other health workers with a systematic guide through the epidemiology, pathophysiology, diagnosis and treatment of angina. We use a question and answer format, and we hope that you find this book a useful and interesting introduction to ischaemic heart disease.

Acknowledgements

We would like to thank the medical editors at Harcourt Health Communications, the publishers; but most of all our many friends and colleagues, the authors, who have given their time to share their skills.

Henry Purcell
Sam Kaddoura
2001

MOSBY
An imprint of Mosby International Limited.

ISBN 0-7234-3255-4

Cataloguing in Publication Data
Catalogue records for this book are available from the US Library of Congress and the British Library.

Note
Medical knowledge is constantly changing. As new information becomes available, changes in treatment, procedures, equipment and the use of drugs become necessary. The editors/authors/contributors and the publishers have taken care to ensure that the information given in this text is accurate and up to date. However, readers are strongly advised to confirm that the information, especially with regard to drug usage, complies with the latest legislation and standards of practice.

The Publisher's policy is to use **paper manufactured from sustainable forests**

Printed and bound by Grafos, SA Arte Sobre papel, Barcelona, Spain.

Contents

List of Contributors

Constantinos Anagnostopoulos, MD PhD, Consultant and Senior Lecturer in Nuclear Medicine, Department of Radiology, Division of Nuclear Medicine, Chelsea and Westminster Hospital, London

Nick Bellenger, BSc MBBS MRCP, Previously: Research Fellow, Cardiovascular Magnetic Resonance Unit, Royal Brompton Hospital, London

Richard A Best, MA FRCP Edin FCCP, Consultant Cardiologist, Burnley General Hospital, Burnley

Carl Brookes, MA MRCP, Consultant Cardiologist, The North Hampshire Hospital, Hampshire

Michael Chester, MBBS MRCP MD, Senior Lecturer in Cardiology, Director National Refractory Angina Centre, Cardiothoracic Centre and University of Liverpool

Miles Dalby, MBBS BSc MRCP, SpR in Cardiology, St Mary's Hospital, London

Anu Garg, BSc MBBS MRCP, Previously: Research Fellow, Division of Cardiology, Hammersmith Hospital, London

Margot A Gosney, MD FRCP, Senior Lecturer, Geriatric Medicine, University Clinical Department, University of Liverpool, Liverpool

Roger Hall, MB FRCP, Professor of Clinical Cardiology, Hammersmith Hospital, London

Clare Hammond, MB ChB MRCP, Cardiologist, Department of Cardiology, University Hospital Aintree, Liverpool

Michael Henein, MSc PhD FESC FACC, Cardiologist, Cardiac Department, Royal Brompton and Harefield NHS Trust, London

Diana R Holdright MD MRCP BSc, Consultant Cardiologist, Department of Cardiology, The Middlesex Hospital (UCL Hospitals), London

Sam Kaddoura, MRCP, Consultant Cardiologist, Department of Cardiology, Chelsea and Westminster Hospital and Royal Brompton Hospital, London

Robert Kelly, MB MRCPI, Research Fellow and Cardiology Registrar, Department of Clinical Pharmacology and Cardiology, Ninewells Hospital, Dundee

Austin Leach, MBBS FFARCS, Consultant Anaesthetist, Royal University Hospital and Pain Specialist, National Refractory Angina Centre, Liverpool

Dudley Pennell, MD FRCP FESC FACC, Clinical Director, Cardiovascular Magnetic Resonance Unit, Royal Brompton Hospital, London

Henry Purcell, MB PhD, Senior Fellow in Cardiology, Department of Cardiology, Royal Brompton Hospital, London

Allan D Struthers, MD FRCP, Professor of Clinical Pharmacology and Consultant Physician, University of Dundee and Medical School, Ninewells Hospital, Dundee

Christine Wright, SRN, Research Nurse, Department of Cardiology, Royal Brompton and Harefield NHS Trust, London

Han B Xiao, MD PhD, Staff Practitioner in Cardiology, Cardiology Department, Central Middlesex Hospital, London

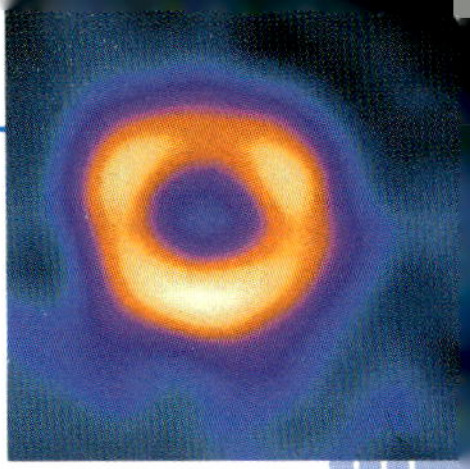

I. Diagnostic Procedures

1. Electrocardiography

Han B Xiao

1. How should the interpretation of an ECG be approached?

An ECG should be interpreted by a doctor who has seen the patient and is fully aware of the clinical context. It is crucial to have good quality recording. Basic ECG measurements including heart rate, PR interval, QRS duration and QT interval are usually measured automatically by a modern electrocardiograph and should be taken into consideration when interpreting the ECG. Apart from these time intervals, the shapes of the P, QRS and ST–T waves, and the relationship of the P waves to the QRS complexes, form the main criteria for ECG analysis. In order to diagnose abnormalities, the doctor needs to be aware of the normal ranges and expected shapes of the ECG deflections, particularly the QRS complexes in different leads.

2. What are typical ECG abnormalities in patients with coronary artery disease?

Patients with coronary heart disease often have a completely normal ECG. When ECG abnormalities are present, however, ST depression represents chronic ischaemia (**Fig. 1.1**), ST elevation represents acute infarction (**Fig. 1.2**), and a pathological Q wave represents myocardial infarction (myocardial death) (**Fig. 1.3**).

3. How does one define ST depression and ST elevation?

An ST depression is defined as when the ST segment shifts downwards ≥1.5 mm below the isoelectric line and does not recover within 80 milliseconds (this is particularly important in exercise ECG). (The PR segment, from the end of the P wave to the onset of the QRS complex, is usually referred to as the isoelectric line.) ST elevation is defined as when the ST segment shifts upwards 1.0 mm (limb leads) or 2.0 mm (chest leads) above the isoelectric line.

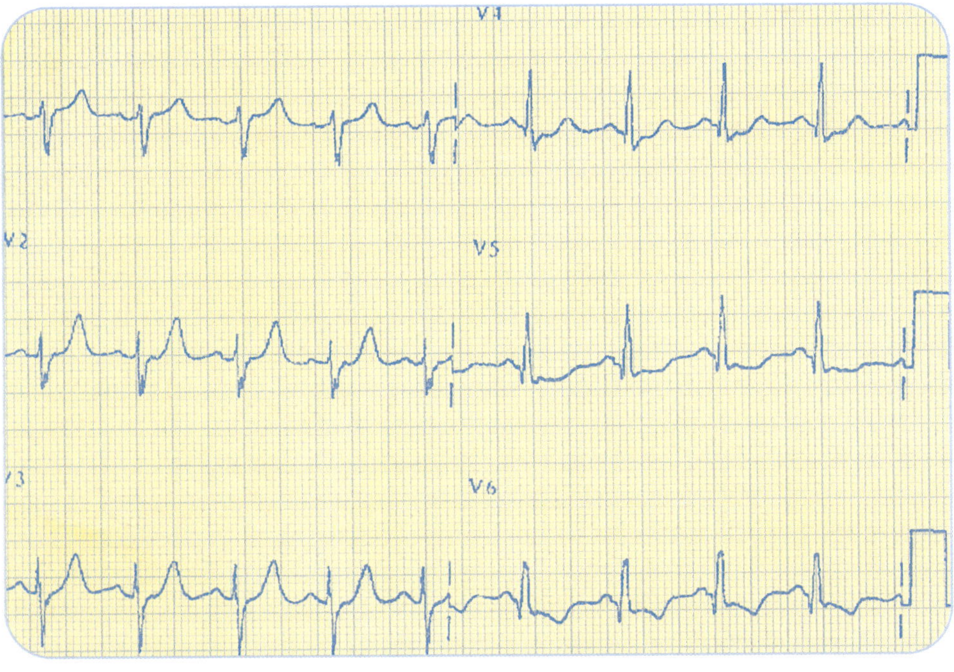

Fig. 1.1 Chest lead ECGs recorded in a patient with recent onset angina demonstrating ST depression in V4 to V6.

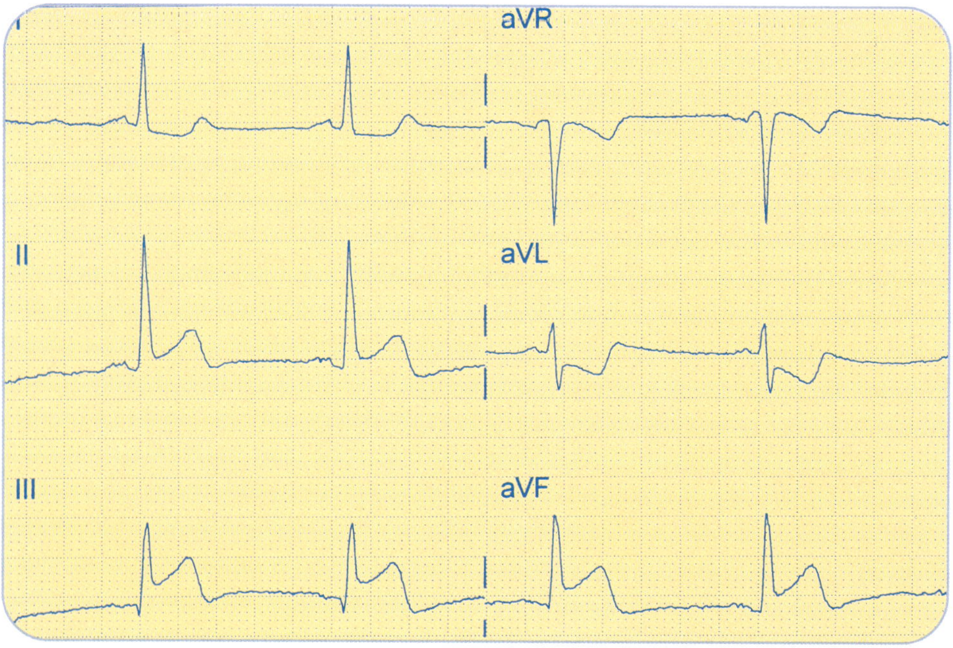

Fig. 1.2 Limb lead ECGs recorded in a patient with an acute myocardial infarction showing ST elevation in II, III and avF.

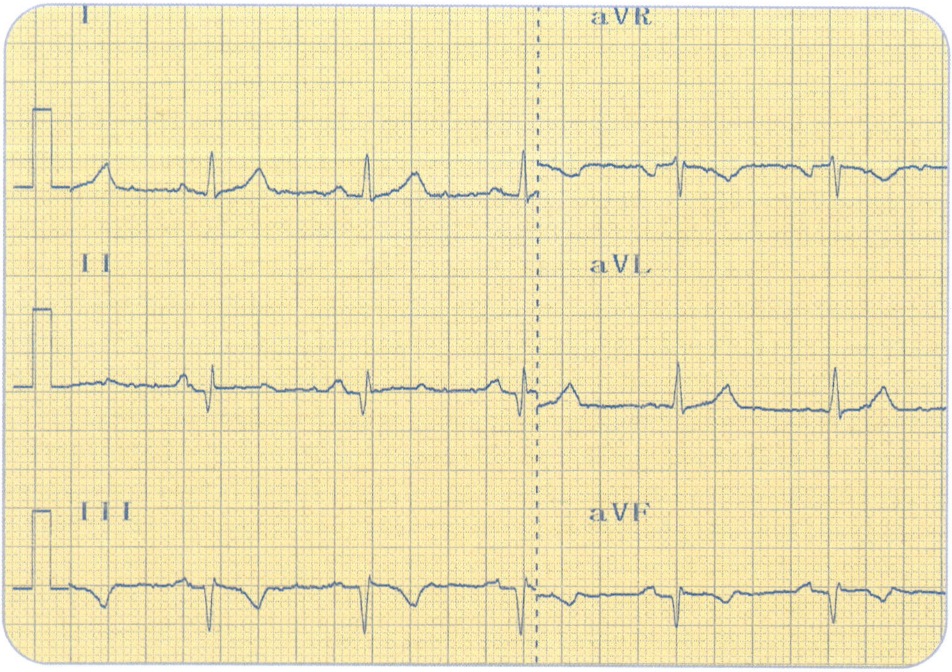

Fig. 1.3 Limb lead ECGs recorded in a patient 3 months after an inferior myocardial infarction showing pathologic Q waves in II, III and avF.

4. What conditions other than coronary artery disease can cause ST depression on a resting ECG?

These include cardiac and non-cardiac pathologies[1].

Cardiac

Cardiomyopathy
Mitral valve prolapse
Severe aortic stenosis
Left ventricular hypertrophy, regardless of cause
Significant volume overload to the left ventricle, e.g. severe mitral and aortic regurgitation
Pre-excitation (WPW) syndrome
Supraventricular tachycardia
Intraventricular conduction defect

Non-cardiac

Anaemia
Hypertension
Glucose load
Hypokalaemia
Hyperventilation
Hypoxia
Digitalis effects

5. What is a pathological Q wave?

A Q wave with a duration of over 40 milliseconds (width = 1 mm) and an amplitude over one-quarter of the total QRS deflection is defined as a pathological Q wave. Q waves (or QS pattern) are often present in lead avR and sometimes V1, but should be considered as abnormal in any other leads.

6. What are the causes of pathological Q waves?

Myocardial infarction is the main cause of pathological Q waves. Other conditions, particularly cardiomyopathies, can also produce pathological Q waves. For example, Q waves in inferior leads can be found in hypertrophic cardiomyopathy, Q waves in anterior leads in dilated cardiomyopathy and left ventricular hypertrophy (e.g. aortic stenosis), and Q waves in all chest leads in amyloid cardiomyopathy. Pathological Q waves in cardiomyopathies can probably be attributed to myocardial fibrosis.

7. What are the early ECG signs of myocardial ischaemia?

In time sequence, inverted T waves, tall and prolonged T waves, and QRS amplitude reduction are the early signs of an acute ischaemic event. All these changes can be readily demonstrated in animal experiments, but are only occasionally seen in humans with unstable angina or in the early stages of acute myocardial infarction. The most commonly seen ECG signs of ischaemia in humans are ST depression and elevation.

8. What is QTc?

QTc is the QT interval corrected for heart rate. QT interval (from the onset of the QRS complex to the end of the T wave) increases with lower heart rates. The correction is made by dividing the QT interval by the square root of the RR interval. The upper limit of normal QTc is 420 milliseconds.

9. What are the commonest causes of QT prolongation?

Myocardial ischaemia, antiarrhythmic drugs and hypocalcaemia.

10. What is a U wave?

A U wave is the deflection after the T wave and before the next P wave. U waves usually point in the same direction as T waves in the same leads. They are best seen in V2 and V3.

11. What is the significance of abnormal U waves?

The most common abnormality is U wave inversion, opposite in direction to the T waves. Inverted (or negative) U waves are usually associated with subendocardial ischaemia in patients with either angina or myocardial infarction as well as severe left ventricular hypertrophy. Inverted U waves are also associated with impaired left ventricular diastolic function in patients with left ventricular hypertrophy.

12. Is ECG able to detect coronary spasm?

Yes. The typical patient with coronary arterial spasm has chest pain or discomfort at rest (variant angina) and normal coronary arteries on subsequent angiography. An ECG recorded during chest pain shows ST elevation, which is sometimes dramatic and resolves completely as chest pain subsides. Other findings include various degrees of A–V block and ventricular ectopics.

13. Can an ECG provide information on the anatomic site of coronary artery disease?

Yes. There is a close relationship between ECG leads where ischaemic abnormalities are found and the anatomic territory of coronary lesions. Ischaemia in the anterior leads, V1 to V3, represents left anterior descending artery disease; in inferior leads, II, III and avF, it represents right or circumflex coronary artery disease; ischaemia in left lateral leads, V4 to V6 or high lateral leads, avL and I, is more ambiguous and can arise in left anterior descending artery disease, diagonal and circumflex coronary artery disease or even right coronary artery disease[1].

14. Are there other ECG measurements for myocardial ischaemia apart from ST–T changes?

Yes. Recent studies have shown that increased variation of QRS morphology (assessed by the onset of the QRS complex) and increased QT dispersion are associated with myocardial ischaemia. The prevalence of late potentials (signals with low amplitude and high frequency at the end of the QRS complex) on a signal averaged ECG is much higher in patients with angina than in normal controls (23 vs. 7.5%).

15. Can conditions other than cardiac chest pain cause ECG changes?

Yes. Anxiety nervousness can cause reduced T wave amplitude in inferior or left precordial leads. This can be reversed by beta-blockers. Hyperventilation can cause reduced or inverted T waves in leads V5 and V6. This is more common in females than in males.

16. Is a resting ECG useful in assessing chest pain?

Yes. A resting ECG can demonstrate any previous myocardial infarction (Q waves), acute ischaemia during recording (ST elevation) and existing bundle branch block. In addition, patients with ischaemic changes on a resting ECG are likely to have significant coronary artery disease and poor prognosis[2]. Newly developed persistent T wave inversion in leads V1 to V3 may indicate left anterior descending coronary artery disease. The combination of chest pain and left bundle branch block or left ventricular hypertrophy is suggestive of coronary artery disease and reduced left ventricular function. Finally, an appropriately recorded resting ECG is essential before an exercise stress test, which is the most commonly used non-invasive method for investigating patients with chest pain. Thus, a resting ECG can provide very useful information on the current status of myocardial ischaemia and cardiac function, further management and prognostic assessment.

17. What are the limitations of a resting ECG in coronary artery disease?

As a resting ECG is a single brief sample and ischaemia is a dynamic event, it is understandable that a resting ECG may be completely normal in patients with coronary artery disease when they are asymptomatic. ECG interpretation is observer dependent and needs to be combined with clinical information. Its sensitivity and specificity are imperfect.

References

1. Fisch C. Electrocardiography. In: Braunwald E (ed.): *Heart Disease. A Textbook of Cardiovascular Medicine*. Philadelphia: WB Saunders Company, 1997:108–52.
2. Gorgels AP, Vos MA, Mulleneers R, *et al.* Value of the electrocardiogram in diagnosing the number of severely narrowed coronary arteries in resting angina pectoris. *Am J Cardiol* 1993;**72**:999–1003.

2. Exercise Stress Test

Han B Xiao

1. What is the most commonly used method for the exercise stress test?

The standard Bruce treadmill protocol. It begins at a 1.7 mph speed and 10% slope (5 METs; see below) with an increase in both speed and slope every 3 minutes (1 stage = 3 minutes after which workload increases, beginning another stage) up to 5.0 mph and 18% respectively. In older patients or those whose exercise capacity is limited, the Bruce protocol can be modified by two 3-minute warm-up stages at 1.7 mph and 0% slope[1,2].

2. What are the indications for an exercise stress test?

Generally, an exercise stress test can be used in three categories:

1. Diagnosis of coronary artery disease

Patients with exertional symptoms, chest pain or dyspnoea
Patients with atypical symptoms
Women with both typical and atypical chest pain

2. Assessment of functional capacity

Patients with stable angina or after myocardial infarction
Patients with valvular disease
Assessment of blood pressure during exercise in patients with treated hypertension who wish to engage in dynamic exercise

3. Assessment of prognosis

Patients with angiographically confirmed coronary artery disease
Patients who have recovered from acute myocardial infarction.

3. What are absolute contraindications for an exercise stress test?

Ongoing acute myocardial ischaemia
Unstable angina
Very high blood pressure, systolic pressure ≥250 mmHg or diastolic pressure ≥120 mmHg
Myocarditis
Pericarditis
Severe aortic stenosis
Any acute systemic illness.

4. Is there a role for the exercise stress test in screening for coronary artery disease?

Yes, but only in special cases. It has been used to screen coronary artery disease in special occupations such as pilots and heavy duty vehicle drivers. Occasionally, it is also used to assess asymptomatic patients who have multiple risk factors for coronary artery disease. In these groups there is a high prevalence of false positive tests.

5. What are the chances of occurrence of the risks associated with an exercise stress test?

Very small. Serious complications such as exercise provoked myocardial infarction or life-threatening arrhythmias are reported in less than 5 per 10,000 (0.05%) tests, and death in less than 1 per 10,000 (0.01%).

6. What patient preparations are necessary before an exercise stress test?

Ideally, patients should discontinue beta-blockers before the test as beta-blockers limit chronotropic response to exercise and increase the chances of false negative results. Patients should also be told what the test entails, why it is required, and warned about possible false positive and negative results. They should wear clothing and shoes suitable for jogging.

7. What non-cardiac conditions may limit the exercise test?

Chronic obstructive airway disease
Severe obesity
Peripheral vascular disease
Arthritis
Any inability to walk on a treadmill regardless of cause

These are not definite contraindications for the test, but limit exercise capacity and impair the usefulness of the test. Patients with such conditions could have alternative approaches to the investigation of inducible myocardial ischaemia, such as nuclear imaging and stress echocardiography.

8. What is a 'maximal predicted heart rate'?

It is the target heart rate that is set for each individual patient. There is usually little to be gained in exercising patients beyond this point as the test becomes unreliable. It varies with age, gender and lifestyle. The simplest and most practical method to estimate the maximal predicted heart rate (MPHR) in an average individual is to use the following formulas:

Male	MPHR = 220 – age (years).
Female	MPHR = 215 – age (years).

9. What is a 'submaximal exercise test'?

Occasionally, patients are deliberately exercised to a lower level heart rate. This test is used in patients who have had a recent myocardial infarction as part of pre-discharge assessment. The aim would be for them to achieve 70–80% maximal predicted heart rate.

10. What is an 'MET'?

MET is the 'metabolic equivalent'. One MET is the amount of oxygen (O_2) consumed per minute by an average subject at rest, approximately 3.5 ml O_2/kg/minute. It is estimated that a minimum of 5 METs are required for carrying out daily activities. The workload of walking on a 10% slope at a speed of 1.7 mph is also 5 METs.

11. What are normal ECG changes during an exercise stress test?

In normal subjects, as heart rate and blood pressure increase with exercise, PR interval and QRS duration both shorten. QRS complex and T wave amplitude may reduce slightly. In addition, it is not uncommon to see up-sloping ST depression (J point depression), which recovers to baseline within 80 milliseconds.

12. What abnormalities on pre-test ECG may make it difficult to interpret an exercise ECG?

Left ventricular hypertrophy
Left or right bundle branch block
ST–T abnormalities
Digitalis effects
Pre-excitation (WPW) syndrome

However, in patients with the above ECG abnormalities, an exercise stress test can still provide useful information on exercise capacity, symptoms, arrhythmias, and heart rate and blood pressure response.

13. What defines a positive exercise test?

1 Horizontal or down-sloping ST depression over 1.5 mm.
2 Up-sloping ST depression over 1.5 mm that does not recover back to baseline at 80 milliseconds.
3 Progressive decline in blood pressure during exercise.

However, there are other ECG changes that should be considered potentially positive even in the absence of ST depression. They include significant increase in QRS duration, the development of left or right bundle branch block or frequent ventricular ectopics, and tachycardia.

14. When should an exercise stress test be terminated?

The reasons for termination include the following symptoms and ECG abnormalities:
Severe chest pain
Severe fatigue or dyspnoea
Ataxia
Significant fall in heart rate
Significant fall in blood pressure
Blood pressure ≥270/120 mmHg
Development of tachyarrhythmias
Development of complete heart block, or left or right bundle branch block
ST depression ≥3 mm
ST elevation ≥1 mm in leads without pathological Q waves.

15. How is work capacity interpreted from an exercise stress test?

Work capacity is assessed by the peak amount of work performed (METs) or exercise stage achieved. Maximal work capacity is affected by other non-pathological factors, including familiarisation with the exercise equipment, level of training and environmental conditions of the test. All these may should be considered when the test is interpreted.

The work capacity is used as a prognostic measurement. In patients with coronary artery disease, a limited exercise capacity (e.g. workload <7 METs, and rate-pressure product <25 mmHg.beat/minute.10^{-3}) is associated with increased cardiac events and worsened prognosis.

16. How useful is an exercise stress test in diagnosing coronary artery disease?

Despite its limitations, coronary angiography is still widely accepted as the gold standard for the diagnosis of coronary artery disease. Using coronary angiography as a standard, an exercise stress test has an overall 70% sensitivity and specificity. In single vessel disease, it has a mean sensitivity of 68% (range: 23 to 100%) and a mean specificity of 77% (range: 17 to 100%). In two vessel disease, it has a mean sensitivity of 81% (range: 40 to 100%) and a mean specificity of 66% (range: 17 to 100%). In triple vessel disease or left anterior descending coronary artery lesion, it has the highest sensitivity (86±11%) but lowest specificity (53±24%).

17. Are the sensitivity and specificity of the exercise test affected by intervention (stent or PTCA)?

No. The mean sensitivity and specificity against coronary angiography are 72 and 77% respectively in patients who have developed ischaemic symptoms after coronary intervention[3].

18. Are there differences between males and females in exercise test?

Yes. False positive results are more common in females than in males and reduce the diagnostic accuracy in female patients. The explanation is that women tend to release more catecholamines during exercise, which may cause coronary vasoconstriction and increase the incidence of ECG changes.

19. What does exercise induced ST elevation imply?

In general, ST elevation represents acute ischaemia or myocardial infarction. During exercise, ST elevation occurring in leads where there are pathological Q waves is associated with resting wall motion abnormalities and low ejection fraction. ST elevation in the absence of Q waves is suggestive of myocardial infarction due to coronary artery spasm or occlusion (found in 1% of patients with severe coronary artery disease).

20. Apart from ST–T changes during exercise, are there any other ECG changes suggestive of myocardial ischaemia?

Yes. Increased R wave amplitude, prolonged QRS duration, lengthened QT interval and increased QT dispersion during exercise are all signs of inducible ischaemia.

21. What does normalisation of inverted T waves during exercise indicate in patients with recovered myocardial infarction?

Viability of the myocardium. It is particularly so in patients who do not have chest pain or ST depression or elevation on resting ECG. It is not uncommon to see an inverted T wave become normal in patients who had no history of myocardial infarction. These patients are usually young and have normal exercise capacity.

22. Can an exercise stress test predict multivessel coronary artery disease and adverse prognosis?

Yes. The following are associated with multivessel disease or adverse prognosis:

1. Symptoms, e.g. chest pain or dyspnoea limited workload (<6 METs).
2. Blood pressure failing to increase (systolic blood pressure ≤140 mmHg) or sustaining at or below resting level during progressive exercise.
3. Heart rate not reaching 120 beats/minute during exercise (in patients who are not on beta-blockers).
4. ST depression ≥2 mm, particularly down-sloping ST depression occurring before 6 METs.
5. ST depression present in ≥5 leads.
6. ST depression persisting for ≥5 minutes into recovery period.
7. ST elevation.
8. Reproducible sustained (>30 seconds) or symptomatic ventricular tachycardia.

References

1. Ellestad MH, Cooke BMJr, Greenberg PS. Stress testing: clinical application and predictive capacity. *Prog Cardiovasc Dis* 1979;**21**:431–60.
2. Chaitman BR: Exercise stress testing. In: Braunwald E (ed.): *Heart Disease. A Textbook of Cardiovascular Medicine*. Philadelphia: WB Saunders Company, 1997;153–76.
3. Legrand V, Rasskinet B, Laarman G, *et al*. Diagnositic value of exercise electrocardiography and angina after coronary artery stenting. Benestent Study Group. *Am Heart J* 1997;**133**:240–8.

3. Holter Monitoring and the Signal-Averaged ECG in Assessment of Myocardial Ischaemia

Christine Wright

1. When was Holter monitoring first used to evaluate ischaemia?

The association between ST segment deviation and angina using ambulatory monitoring was first described by Holter in 1961. He went on to develop a series of recorders to evaluate the ECG in ambulant patients[1]. There were concerns that the devices used initially had poor frequency responses which might distort the ST segment. However, over the next 10 years, frequency modulated devices became available, such that the use of Holter monitoring to detect myocardial ischaemia increased dramatically.

During the seventies and eighties there was an explosion of interest in using ambulatory monitoring to study the patterns of ST segment changes in patients with stable and unstable coronary syndromes and Prinzmetal's angina. It soon became apparent that the majority of episodes of ST segment depression were asymptomatic and had similar characteristics in terms of heart rate rise and duration to those episodes accompanied by angina. Treatment should therefore be aimed at the elimination of painful ischaemia as this will have the same effect on silent ischaemia[2].

2. Is there any prognostic benefit in assessment of ambulatory myocardial ischaemia?

The terms 'silent myocardial ischaemia' and 'total ischaemic burden' were introduced, and many studies were undertaken to examine the clinical significance of silent myocardial ischaemia and to determine whether it had any prognostic implications. Silent myocardial ischaemia has been confirmed as representing true ischaemia in patients with coronary artery disease. Studies have shown differing outcomes depending on patient selection. The general conclusion is that the greater the number of episodes of silent and painful ischaemia the more severe the coronary disease. As similar information can be obtained from an exercise test, little further knowledge can be obtained from Holter monitoring and it does not have a role in the routine assessment and management of patients with coronary artery disease[3].

There appears to be no prognostic value in the detection of transient ischaemia in patients with chronic stable angina[4]. Mulcahy *et al*. followed up 221 patients with proven coronary artery disease over a period of four years; each patient had several non-invasive tests including ambulatory monitoring as well as a coronary angiogram. They found that none of the non-invasive tests was of prognostic significance. The only significant independent predictor was the number of vessels diseased.

3. What is the role of Holter monitoring in unstable angina?

Ambulatory monitoring has also been used in acute coronary syndromes. Studies have shown that in patients with unstable angina, ST segment depression on continuous monitoring is a powerful predictor of adverse outcome even if the 12 lead ECG is normal[5]. Patel *et al*. concluded that continuous ST segment monitoring is very useful in identifying high risk subsets of patients soon after admission who may benefit from early intervention.

4. Is there a role for Holter monitoring in myocardial infarction?

It is common practice for post-myocardial infarction patients to have a sub-maximal exercise test prior to discharge to help evaluate the presence of myocardial ischaemia and identify those who might benefit from early revascularisation. It is estimated that 30% of patients undergoing exercise testing post-myocardial infarction have a positive exercise test. Mortality in this group may be as high as 27%; however, a substantial group of patients are unable to exercise, including those at high risk of a coronary event. It has also been shown that a submaximal test may be less predictive than maximal stress testing performed later[6]. Gill found that myocardial ischaemia detected by ambulatory monitoring is common early after acute myocardial infarction and provides further prognostic information even if the exercise test is negative. Indeed, a positive Holter recording showed that the risk of an adverse event was more than doubled[7].

5. What are the benefits and limitations of Holter monitoring?

Ambulatory monitoring is, of course, invaluable in diagnosing atrial and ventricular arrhythmias commonly found in the ischaemic patient. Holter monitoring of the ST segment has been most commonly used in the investigation of patients with chest pain which occurs primarily at rest, in whom exercise testing is negative or where the patient is unable to exercise. It should be remembered that drugs such as digoxin can distort the ST segment and that ST analysis should be avoided if the ECG shows configurations such as left bundle branch block or left ventricular hypertrophy.

Holter monitoring for ischaemia is most commonly used in pharmaceutical trials to evaluate the efficacy of new products, which are usually compared with placebo.

Most modern Holter systems have a low enough frequency response to accurately measure ST segment changes. All tapes should be calibrated for ST analysis and it has been found that 48 hours of recording is the optimum amount of time to detect myocardial ischaemia in everyday life.

Solid state devices have also been evaluated and many are considered suitable for use in ST segment monitoring[8].

6. How is a Holter recorder applied?

The most important aspect of a good quality 24-hour tape is skin preparation. The aim is to reduce the skin impedance so that artefact from muscle movement is diminished as much as possible. The areas where the electrodes are to be placed should be prepared by shaving if necessary and cleaning the site. They should then be abraded until red, and dried thoroughly. The recommended lead positions are shown in **Fig. 3.1**.

The CM5 lead is a bipolar lead which is similar to the V5 on the surface ECG. It has been found to be to be reliable for detecting myocardial ischaemia mainly in the anterior region of the heart[9]. Most recorders have two channels and a good choice for the second channel is an inferior lead such as a modified lead II; some centres prefer to use a modified lead V2 for arrhythmia detection.

The ECG can sometimes change in configuration (when the patient lies flat for example). This postural change can be misleading for analysis. The patient should be asked to lie flat so that any postural changes can be noted and taken into account during the tape analysis.

The patient should be given an angina diary so that episodes can be identified as painful or silent. As the equipment is quite specialised and expensive it is probably not suitable for primary care groups, although application of the Holter tapes could be done at the GP surgery and the cassette posted to the cardiac centre for analysis.

7. How are Holter tapes analysed for ST segment changes?

Most modern Holter systems offer ST segment analysis, using a series of reference dots between the P and Q waves, on the J point, and 80 milliseconds from the J to monitor the ST segment, and compressing the analysis into a 24-hour trend (**Fig. 3.2**).

Conventionally, an ischaemic episode follows the '1 x 1 x 1' rule, where the depression lasts for one minute or more, is separated by one minute from the previous episode, and is one millimetre of ST depression 80 milliseconds from the J point.

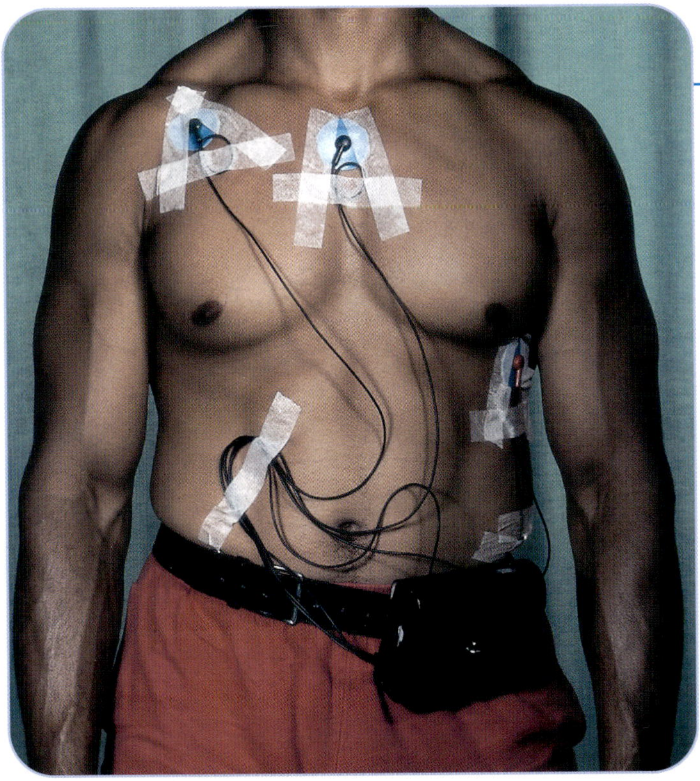

Fig. 3.1
Photograph showing lead positions: CM5 (manubrium and V5) Modified lead II (right shoulder and left iliac crest).

Occasionally ST segment elevation can be detected and this is associated with coronary artery spasm or an evolving myocardial infarction. The tape should be analysed manually to eliminate artefact which can masquerade as ST shift on the trend or automatic final report. The trend should be used to examine where any episodes may have been missed. Strips of ECG at the beginning of the episode should be played out to measure the heart rate and at the point where the maximum amount of ST depression has occurred so that this can be measured. The tape should also be analysed for any arrhythmias and whether they are associated with ischaemia.

8. What is a 'signal-averaged ECG'?

Signal averaging is a process of ECG acquisition that will allow the ECG to be digitised, amplified and analysed to microvolt size potentials. It has been long established that late potentials (i.e. at the end of the QRS) are present in people with coronary artery disease recovering from myocardial infarction and prone to ventricular arrhythmias.

The predictive value of late potentials will depend on the criteria used in defining a late potential[10]. These tiny potentials would normally be obscured by the low signal-to-noise ratio. Thus, the process of acquiring a template of the normal signal is used for comparison by all consecutive beats. A large number of beats are acquired until the signal-to-noise ratio is at an appropriate level (0.3 microvolts). It is these that are used to create the final signal-averaged ECG (SAECG).

The lead system for signal averaging is the XYZ (Frank lead system). The noise on an ECG is random and thus can be eliminated by averaging between 100 to 500 beats.

The most important measurement of SAECG is the QRS duration, which can be measured manually if required. Late potentials cause the QRS to be longer than normal. Late potentials are usually defined as the potentials present in the last 40 milliseconds of the QRS vector and should be below the 40 microvolt threshold (low amplitude signals).

9. When is it useful to use signal-averaged ECG?

SAECG is useful in stratifying patients at risk of sustained ventricular arrhythmias such as those recovering from myocardial infarction. The ECG should be sinus rhythm without bundle branch block or intraventricular conduction delay. SAECG is also useful for identifying patients with ischaemic heart disease and unexplained syncope who could have inducible sustained ventricular tachycardia. It is not recommended for patients with ischaemic heart disease and documented sustained ventricular arrhythmias, or in asymptomatic patients without detectable heart disease[11].

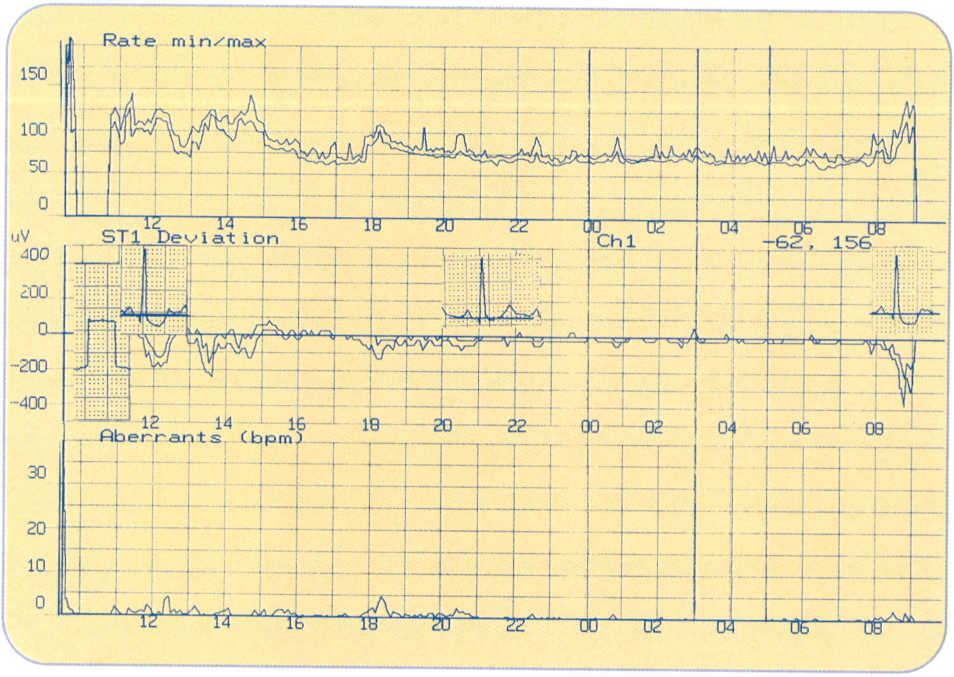

Fig. 3.2 Twenty-four hour trend showing the heart rate and ST deviation.

References

1. Holter N. New method for heart studies with continuous electrocardiography of active subjects. *Science* 1962;**134**:1214–20.
2. Mulcahy D, Keegan J, Fox K, *et al*. Characteristics of silent and painful ischaemia during ambulatory monitoring in patients with coronary arterial disease. *Int J Cardiol* 1990;**28**:377–9.
3. Mulcahy D, Purcell H, Fox K, *et al*. Detection of ambulatory ischaemia is not of practical clinical value in the routine management of patients with stable angina. *Eur Heart J* 1995;**16**:317–24.
4. Mulcahy D, Geller N, Quyyumi A, *et al*. Ischemia during ambulatory monitoring as a prognostic indicator in patients with stable coronary artery disease. *J Am Med Assoc* 1997;**277**:318–24.
5. Patel D, Purcell H, Fox K. Early continuous ST segment monitoring in unstable angina: prognostic value additional to the clinical characteristics and the admission electrocardiogram. *Heart* 1996;**75**:222–8.
6. Juneau M, Colles P, Theroux P, *et al*. Symptom limited versus low level exercise testing before hospital discharge after myocardial infarction. *J Am Coll Cardiol* 1992;**20**:927–33.
7. Gill J, Tomlinson C, Gent M, *et al*. Prognostic importance of myocardial ischaemia detected by ambulatory monitoring early after acute myocardial infarction. *N Eng J Med* 1996;**334**:65–70.
8. Phadke K, Mulcahy D, Fox K. Clinical validation of four solid state ambulatory monitoring devices in detecting shift of the ST segment. *Int J Cardiol* 1991;**33**:445–6.
9. Quyyumi AA, Crake T, Mockus LJ, *et al*. Value of the bipolar lead CM5 in electrocardiography. *Br Heart J* 1986;**56**:372–6.
10. ESC, AHA, ACC. Policy Statement: Standards for analysis of ventricular late potentials using high resolution of signal averaged electrocardiography. *Circulation* 1991;**83**:1481–8.
11. ACC. Expert consensus document SAECG. *J Am Coll Cardiol* 1996;**27(1)**:238–49

4. Echocardiography in Angina Pectoris

Michael Henein

1. What is the role of echocardiography in the investigation of angina pectoris?

Once the possibility of angina pectoris arises from the history, the standard pathway of investigation includes resting ECG, exercise stress test, and, if clinically warranted, coronary arteriography. This policy is in line with recent guidelines for the management of patients with chronic stable angina[1]. Echocardiography may impinge on this diagnostic cascade at a number of points. It must be remembered that coronary artery disease, although much the most common cause of angina pectoris in Western society, is by no means the only one. Angina may be the presenting symptom of valvular aortic stenosis or hypertrophic cardiomyopathy, two conditions that can be very reliably diagnosed by resting echocardiography. Another condition that may mimic angina pectoris is the pain associated with dilatation of the ascending aorta. This is characteristically aggravated by exercise and relieved by rest. Again, aortic dilatation can be recognised by echocardiography. Echocardiography, either transthoracic or transoesophageal, has little place in the study of coronary artery disease itself. However, it is an excellent means of quantifying the nature and extent of ventricular involvement that may be present in patients with angina pectoris due to coronary artery disease. Finally, stress echocardiography has emerged as a very important means of assessing the physiological importance of the coronary artery stenoses demonstrated at angiography.

2. What is the role of transthoracic echocardiography?

Left ventricular disease

After excluding structural cardiac abnormalities as possible causes for angina, coronary artery disease remains the most common cause. In the majority of cases with previous myocardial infarction, transthoracic two-dimensional echocardiography shows obvious wall motion abnormalities. The loss of myocardial tissue is indicative of scar formation; when the myocardium decreases in total thickness the muscle is irreversibly damaged[2]. With massive anteroapical infarction, an apical aneurysm may develop which can easily be diagnosed by its characteristic dyskinetic behaviour in systole. In the absence of prior infarction, resting left ventricular wall motion may be entirely normal as shown by both two-dimensional images and M-mode. Segmental hypokinesis develops as the disease progresses. Other systemic diseases, i.e. hypertension and diabetes, are commonly associated with coronary artery disease. In the former the left ventricle is often hypertrophied and in both, thinning rate of its free wall reduced[3]. With further disease progression, left ventricular systolic function deteriorates, as shown by falling ejection or shortening fraction, and its filling pressures rise, predisposing to subendocardial ischaemia. Doppler demonstrates the typical transmitral 'restrictive physiology' pattern with a dominant E wave, a shortened deceleration time and reduced or absent A wave[4].

Recently, the component of longitudinal ventricular function, termed 'ventricular long axis', which represents the subendocardial layer of the myocardium, has attracted the interest of cardiologists, particularly in the presence of coronary artery disease. It demonstrates longitudinal behaviour, mainly that of the basal part (**Fig. 4.1**), of the left ventricle when it moves towards and away from the ventricular apex in systole and diastole, respectively[5]. It has proved sensitive in demonstrating significant disturbances in patients with coronary artery disease at rest, in spite of the absence of symptoms. The anteroseptal long axis is always abnormal in left anterior descending artery disease (**Fig. 4.2**), and the posterior and right ventricular free wall long axis in right coronary artery disease[6]. In these patients, ventricular long axis function in systole may be completely normal whereas diastolic function is commonly disturbed, showing delayed onset of lengthening and reduced lengthening velocity. These resting abnormalities tend to normalise within 48 hours of successful coronary angioplasty[7]. In addition, these abnormalities, even though they are recorded at rest and in the absence of symptoms, have been shown to be sensitive enough to predict stress induced myocardial perfusion abnormalities shown by thallium scanning. Systolic long axis disturbances correlate with fixed and diastolic ones with reversible perfusion defects[8]. Left ventricular hypertrophy makes the picture difficult to interpret, since it produces similar disturbances to those of coronary artery disease[9].

Pulsed wave Doppler

There is no specific left ventricular filling pattern, at rest, in patients with angina. With progression of left ventricular disease early diastolic relaxation becomes incoordinate causing the rate of pressure fall to drop, so that diastolic filling is compromised, and late diastolic filling becomes dominant[10] (**Fig. 4.3**). This is a non-specific finding since it appears with age as well as with other ventricular diseases. As described above, a high left atrial pressure causes a restrictive filling pattern, regardless of any relaxation abnormality that may present[11]. With stress echocardiography filling pattern changes as wall motion disturbances appear. These are secondary changes, and should not be taken on their own as markers of angina.

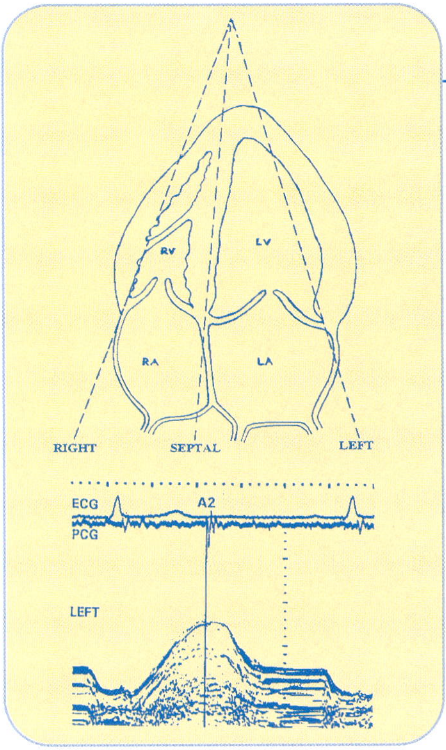

Fig. 4.1
Top: apical 4 chamber view showing the M-mode cursor positioned at the left and septal angles of the mitral ring and the lateral angle of the tricuspid ring. Bottom: M-mode recording from a normal subject taken from the left site of the mitral ring. ECG, electrocardiogram; PCG, phonocardiogram.

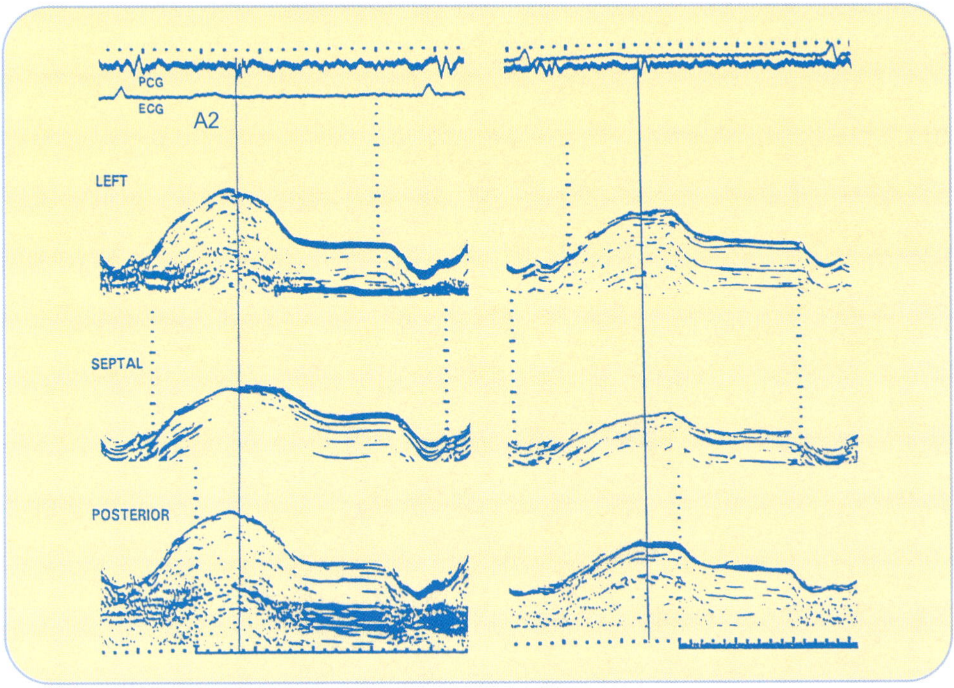

Fig. 4.2 Left, septal and posterior long axes from a patient with isolated left anterior descending artery stenosis (left) and another with anterior myocardial infarction (right). Note the delayed onset of lengthening and reduced lengthening velocity at the septal site in the absence of prior infarction, and the significant fall in total excursion after infarction.

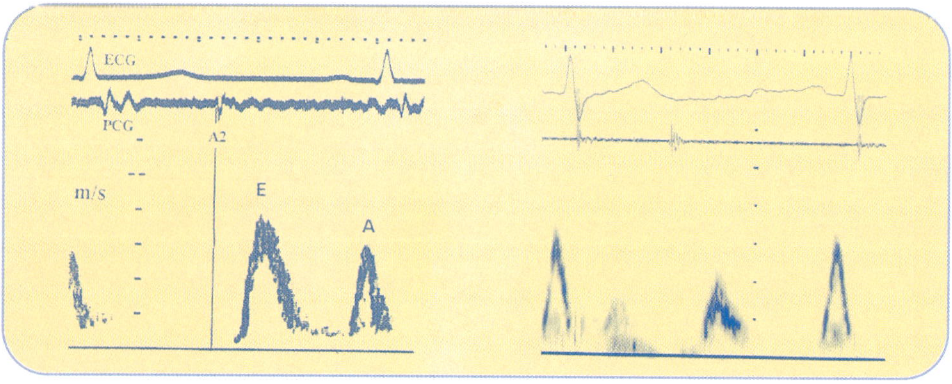

Fig. 4.3 Transmitral Doppler flow velocities from a normal subject (left) and a patient with left ventricular disease (right). Note the development of dominant late diastolic filling component with disease.

Continuous wave Doppler

Like pulsed wave, continuous wave Doppler has no direct role in the diagnosis of angina. It may show mild mitral regurgitation due to papillary muscle dysfunction. However, with significant left ventricular disease functional mitral regurgitation could vary from mild to severe. With prior free wall infarction organic mitral regurgitation might be found due to posterior mitral leaflet prolapse.

Colour Doppler:

Colour Doppler technique is useful for assessing valve disease, particularly regurgitation as well as intracardiac shunts, i.e. ASD and VSD. In patients with coronary artery disease, however, its overall contribution is small, though it may show mitral regurgitation resulting from significant papillary muscle dysfunction.

Tissue Doppler

This is a recently developed technique that demonstrates segmental myocardial behaviour during the cardiac cycle. It delineates the inward and outward movement of the myocardium in systole and diastole in colour. Thus, it may perhaps add to the clarification of the abnormalities previously seen by standard M-mode[12]. A clear understanding of the disturbances detected by the gray scale is essential in interpreting tissue Doppler images. When in the pulsed wave mode it can be used to assess shortening and lengthening segmental velocities. Its main limitation, however, is that it does not allow for the assessment of amplitude or timing of different segments. It therefore should not be used in isolation, but the information it gives may be useful when combined with other echocardiography techniques.

3. Is there a role for routine trans-oesophageal echocardiography (TOE) in assessment of angina pectoris?

Routine TOE has no role in preoperative assessment of patients with angina, since ventricular function is poorly studied from the back of the heart; this can instead easily and clearly be studied with transthoracic echocardiography. However, it has significant value when used intraoperatively, during coronary artery surgery, bypass, and minimal or beating heart surgery[13]. It has shown early recovery of ventricular function in beating heart surgery compared to bypass surgery that correlates with the differences in myocardial injury and troponin concentration in the two conditions[14]. Although the use of intraoperative TOE has been primarily for research purposes, it has increasingly been used for routine monitoring of cardiac surgery. It can demonstrate the consequences of early graft occlusion soon after surgery as well as during the early postoperative period, as shown by wall motion disturbances, at a time when reoperation is feasible and extensive myocardial infarction avoidable.

4. How sensitive is echocardiography in determining wall motion abnormalities?

Ventricular wall motion abnormalities resulting from coronary artery disease have been intensively studied using contrast angiography. The onset of systole may be locally delayed and the whole period of systole prolonged. Thus, the end of systole becomes asynchronous in the cavity resulting in early diastole being incoordinate[15]. Two-dimensional echocardiography, although commonly obtained at different views to ventriculograms, has proved a satisfactory means for detecting regional abnormalities in the amplitude of wall motion in these patients. This is more evident when disturbances are severe and localised, as occurs after myocardial infarction[16]. Its sensitivity in detecting contrast angiographic wall movement abnormalities has increased over the years with the progressive improvement in image resolution and hence delineation of endocardial border. It has approached 96% for normal segments and 93% for dysfunctional ones, i.e. showing akinesis or dyskinesis[17]. The accuracy of this subjective assessment depends on determining segments outside the 95% confidence limit of normal. The latter themselves are difficult to determine[18]. In addition, the presence of other commonly associated diseases; such as hypertension and diabetes, may influence ventricular function and the overall wall motion score. Therefore, wall motion assessment in these conditions needs careful analysis, including other parameters in addition to the simple amplitude of movement. Because of the known limitations of two-dimensional echocardiograms for applying time and velocity changes in its analysis, M-mode, with its slow repetition rate, has proved ideal in this respect. When obtained with high strip speed details of amplitude, time and velocity can be documented and abnormalities outside the normal range identified. Indeed, resting left ventricular long axis disturbances, as detected by M-mode echocardiography, has shown 90% sensitivity and 87% specificity in detecting stress induced reversible perfusion defects, shown by thallium scanning in patients with coronary artery disease in the absence of prior myocardial infarction[8].

5. What are the advantages of stress echocardiography?

The combination of standard ECG and echocardiography at peak exercise for determining wall motion abnormalities in patients with angina has been used to identify stress induced wall motion disturbances as a marker of coronary insufficiency[19]. However, it is difficult to get echocardiographic images at peak exercise. In recent years, therefore, pharmacological stress echocardiography has been applied, using different agents, e.g. adenosine[20], dipyridamole, and more recently dobutamine[21]. The latter has become a routine test. Again, standard stress echocardiography involves semi-quantitative analysis of two-dimensional echocardiographic images of left ventricular short and long axes taken from different views. A positive test is based on identifying new wall motion disturbances – hypokinesia, akinesia or even dyskinesia. A cumulative wall motion score taken from different views is used to assess the extent of stress induced wall motion disturbances secondary to coronary artery disease. This technique can be used to identify ischaemic, hibernating and scarred segments according to their response to the positive inotropic agent with different doses. It has been shown to be useful in assessing the beneficial effect of surgical and non-surgical coronary revascularisation in exertional angina due to significant coronary artery disease, and to assess surgical risk[22]. It has similar sensitivity and specificity to thallium perfusion imaging in identifying reversible ischaemia[23].

Ventricular long axis function studied during dobutamine stress echocardiography is also useful in diagnosis of exertional angina, particularly when combined with phonocardiogram. It has proved sensitive in demonstrating wall motion disturbances similar to the resting ones, both in systole and diastole[24]. Systolic abnormalities correlate with abnormal stress induced ventricular depolarisation and diastolic abnormalities with delayed repolarisation. The technique can show similar disturbances in right ventricular behaviour at peak stress which suggest right ventricular ischaemia, particularly in patients with right coronary artery disease, a difficult diagnosis to make by other methods. Findings in individual cases have confirmed the sensitivity of long axis abnormalities in detecting ventricular dysfunction resulting from subclinical coronary artery disease and also stress induced coronary spasm[25].

6. What are the other indications for stress echocardiography?

In addition to the useful application of stress echocardiography in coronary artery disease it has proved particularly useful, in combination with continuous wave Doppler, in identifying abnormalities other than those of wall motion, as possible causes of exertional symptoms. In elderly patients with exertional shortness of breath and chest pain and normal left ventricular systolic function, stress echocardiography has shown signs of dynamic ventricular outflow tract obstruction, i.e. systolic anterior movement of mitral valve and development of high outflow tract pressure drop[26]. Similar findings have been seen before in patients with hypertrophic cardiomyopathy and exertional symptoms, and to a much lesser extent after non-surgical septal reduction. Again, in the presence of an underestimated aortic stenosis at rest and severe left ventricular disease, stress echocardiography has an important role in differentiating between the two conditions, at high heart rate, as two different mechanisms causing angina. Finally, stress echocardiography can be used in demonstrating stress-induced arrhythmias as well as conduction abnormalities as possible causes of exertional chest discomfort. Thus, it is always advisable that exertional symptoms should be studied during stress rather than at rest.

CONCLUSION

For routine practice of cardiology, transthoracic echocardiography is the technique of choice for excluding structural cardiac causes of angina. Stress echocardiography demonstrates wall motion disturbances due to coronary artery disease, as well as Doppler signs of ventricular outflow tract obstruction in symptomatic patients with left ventricular hypertrophy.

References

1. ACC/AHA/ACP-ASIM. Guidelines for the management of patients with chronic stable angina: executive summary and recommendations. *Circulation* 1999;**99**:2829–48.
2. Rasmussen S, Corya BC, Feigenbaum H, *et al*. Detection of myocardial scar tissue by M-mode echocardiography. *Circulation* 1978;**57**:230.
3. Henein MY, Xiao HB, Brecker SJD, *et al*. Bernheim 'a' wave:obstructed right ventricular inflow or atrial cross talk? *Br Heart J* 1993;**69**:409–13.
4. Appleton CP, Hatle LK, Popp RL. Demonstration of restrictive ventricular physiology by Doppler echocardiography. *J Am Coll Cardiol* 1988;**11**:757–68.
5. Henein MY, Gibson DG. Normal long axis function. *Heart* 1999;**81**:111–13.
6. Henein MY. Ventricular long axis function in coronary artery disease (PhD thesis). London: Imperial College, London University, 1997.
7. Henein MY, Priestley K, Davarashvili T, *et al*. Early changes in left ventricular subendocardial function after successful coronary angioplasty. *Br Heart J* 1993;**69**:501–6.
8. Henein MY, Das SK, O'Sullivan C, *et al*. Left ventricular long axis disturbances as predictors for thallium perfusion defects in coronary artery disease. *Heart* 1998;**79**;295–300.
9. Henein MY, Gibson DG. Suppression of left ventricular early diastolic filling by long axis asynchrony. *Br Heart J* 1995;**73**:151–7.
10. Henein MY, Gibson DG. Abnormal subendocardial function in restrictive left ventricular disease. *Br Heart J* 1994;**72**:237–42.
11. Nagueh SF, Middleton KJ, Kopelen HA, *et al*. Doppler tissue imaging: a noninvasive technique for evaluation of left ventricular relaxation and estimation of filling pressures. *J Am Coll Cardiol*. 1997;**15**:1527–33.
12. Koh TW, Pepper JR, Gibson DG. Early changes in left ventricular anterior wall dynamics and coordination after coronary artery surgery. *Heart* 1997;**78**:291–7.
13. Koh TW, Hooper J, Kemp M, *et al*. Intraoperative release of troponin T in coronary venous and arterial blood and its relation to recovery of left ventricular function and oxidative metabolism following coronary artery surgery. *Heart* 1998;**80**:341–8.
14. Gibson DG, Prewitt TA, Brown DJ. Analysis of left ventricular wall movement during isovolumic relaxation and its relation to coronary artery disease. *Br Heart J* 1976;**38**:1010–19.
15. Ohuchi Y, Kuwako K, Umeda T, *et al*. Real time, phased array cross sectional echocardiographic evaluation of left ventricular asynergy and quantitation of left ventricular function. *Jpn Heart J* 1980;**21**:1–15.
16. Kronik G, Hutterer B, Schmoliner R, *et al*. Sensitivitat und soezifitat der zweidimensionalen echokardiographie bei er diagnose von herzinfarktnarben. *Klin Wochenschr* 1981;**59**:187–95.
17. Marier DL, Gibson DG. Limitations of two frame method for displaying regional left ventricular wall motion inman. *Br Heart J* 1980;**44**:555–9.
18. Ryan T, Vasey CG, Presti CF, *et al*. Exercise echocardiography: detection of coronary artery disease in patients with normal left ventricular wall motion at rest. *J Am Coll Cardiol* 1988;**11**:993–9.
19. Zoghbi W, Cheirif J, Kleiman NS, *et al*. Diagnosis of ischaemic heart disease with adenosine echocardiography. *J Am Coll Cardiol* 1991;**18**:1271–9.
20. Poli A, Previtali M, Lanzarini L, *et al*. Comparison of dobutamine stress echocardiography with dipyridamole stress echocardiography for detection of viable myocardium after myocardial infarction treated with thrombolysis. *Heart* 1996;**75**:240–6.
21. Perrone-Filardi P, Pace L, Prastaro M, *et al*. Dobutamine echocardiography predicts improvement of hypoperfused dysfunctional myocardium after revascularization in patients with coronary artery disease. *Circulation* 1995;**91**:2556–65.
22. Marwick T, D'Hondt A-M, Baudhuin T, *et al*. Optimal use of dobutamine stress for the detection and evaluation of coronary artery disease: combination with echocardiography or scintigraphy, or both? *J Am Coll Cardiol* 1993;**22**:159–67.
23. O'Sullivan C, Henein MY, Sutton R, *et al*. Abnormal ventricular activation and repolarisation during dobutamine stress echocardiography in coronary artery disease. *Heart* 1998;**79**:468–73.
24. Cooke FJ, Clague J, Henein MY. Stress long axis function in coronary artery spasm. *Clin Cardiol* 1999;**22**:757–8.
25. Henein MY, O'Sullivan CA, Coats AJS, *et al*. Stress induced left ventricular outflow tract obstruction – a potential cause of dyspnoea in the elderly. *J Am Coll Cardiol* 1997;**30**:1301–7.
26. Knight C, Kurbaan AS, Seggewiss H, *et al*. Non-surgical septal reduction for hypertrophic obstructive cardiomyopathy: outcome in the first series of patients. *Circulation* 1997;**95**:2075–81.

5. Nuclear Cardiology Testing in Angina Pectoris

Constantinos Anagnostopoulos

1. What radionuclide tests are employed in assessing patients with chest pain?

Diagnostic testing is an important component of cardiovascular medicine. Among the tests used in patients investigated for coronary artery disease (CAD), myocardial perfusion imaging (MPI) has become established as a useful non-invasive method for assessing not only the presence or absence of disease but also its extent and severity. The technique is very simple, involving an injection of MPI agents such as thallium-201- or technetium-99m-labelled tracers at peak exercise or during pharmacological stress and the heart is imaged with a gamma-camera. Images can be either planar or tomographic.

The creation of a perfusion image depends on the ability of the radiotracers to be distributed throughout the myocardium in proportion to regional flow. They distribute uniformly in normally perfused myocardium (**Fig. 5.1**). Inducible myocardial ischaemia or disparities in regional myocardial blood flow cause perfusion defects. Similarly, infarcted areas appear as perfusion defects. Imaging at rest permits reassessment of the defects: defects, which disappear (reversible) indicate inducible hypoperfusion; those that persist (fixed) indicate necrotic myocardium (**Figs 5.2** & **5.3**).

Dynamic exercise is the most usual type of stress but dipyridamole or adenosine[1] (alone or in combination with mild to moderate exercise) is an excellent alternative for patients with suboptimal exercise tolerance. Patients with asthma, or severe obstructive pulmonary disease, who are at risk of developing adverse effects from either adenosine or dipyridamole, can be stressed safely with dobutamine[2].

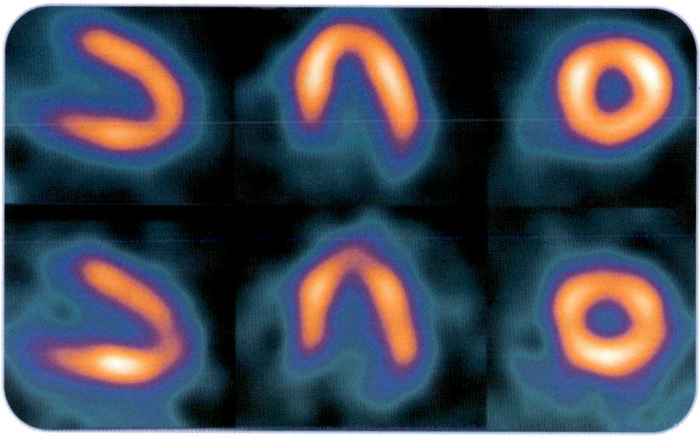

Fig. 5.1
Normal myocardial perfusion tomograms in vertical long axis (left), horizontal long axis (centre) and short axis planes (right).

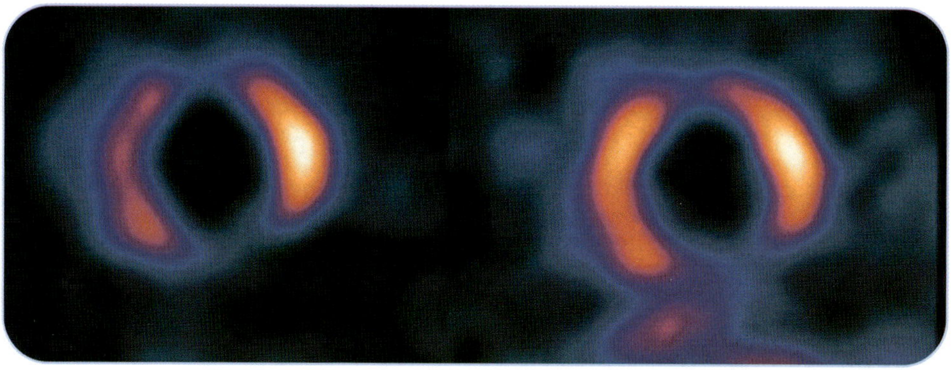

Fig. 5.2 Short axis Tc-99m-MIBI planes, immediately after stress (left) and at rest (right) in a patient with angina and previous inferior myocardial infarction. There is a reversible defect in the septum and a partially reversible defect in the anterior wall, which are both suggestive of inducible ischaemia in the left anterior descending artery. In addition there is a permanent (fixed) defect in the inferior wall indicative of myocardial infarction.

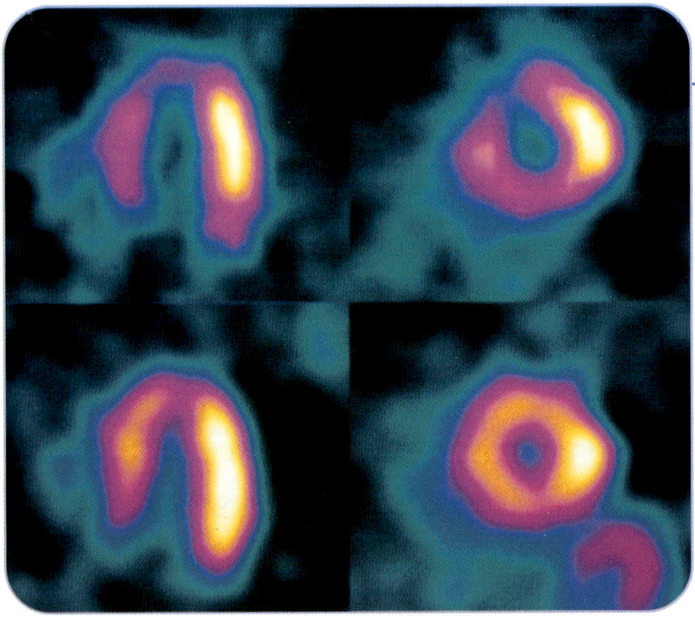

Fig. 5.3
Horizontal (left) and short axis (right) views from a patient with a left anterior descending artery stenosis. The scan shows inducible ischaemia in the anterior wall and septum.

2. What are the differences between thallium-201 and technetium-99m MPI?

Thallium-201 has been used routinely as a tracer of myocardial perfusion for almost two decades. Normal appearances of both planar and tomographic images are well established and the protocols for acquisition and image processing have been standardised.

Thallium-201 is administered intravenously as thallous chloride and the usual dose is 80 MBq. Imaging starts within five to 10 minutes of injection and should be completed within 30 minutes. During this period the distribution of thallium-201 within the myocardium is relatively fixed and, despite the cessation of stress testing, the images reflect myocardial perfusion at peak stress[3]. Thallium-201 then washes out of the myocardium and the rate is slower in hypoperfused than in normally perfused myocardium. In fact, there is an equilibration between the intracellular and intravascular thallium-201, with a continuous extraction and release of thallium-201 by viable myocytes. As a result of the different wash out rates between normal and hypoperfused myocardium, areas with decreased initial uptake will demonstrate improvement of thallium-201 activity 2–4 hours later[4].

This phenomenon of improvement or 'fill-in' of a perfusion defect over time is known as 'redistribution'. The practical consequence of this phenomenon is that the images acquired shortly after injection reflect myocardial perfusion during stress, and those several hours later reflect the distribution of viable myocardium. Comparison between the two sets of images allows distinction between inducible hypoperfusion and myocardial necrosis in the majority of patients, although in some cases, redistribution may be incomplete at four hours and a second thallium-201 injection is needed to differentiate between ischaemia and scarring[5].

Thallium-201 has also been used in several ways for identifying myocardial viability and hibernation. It has been compared with ^{18}F fluoro-deoxyglucose (FDG), a radiotracer used in positron emission tomography (PET) studies and is regarded as the gold standard for assessment of myocardial viability and hibernation. In most cases a reasonable agreement was found between thallium-201 and PET imaging[6].

Thallium-201, however, has some limitations. First, because of the relatively long half-life within the body, radiation exposure to the patient is high. Eighty megabecquerels delivers an effective dose equivalent of 17 mSv and this is more than the average exposure during coronary arteriography. Second, because of the desire to limit radiation exposure, the injected dose is kept low and, to compound the problem, only 4% of the injected dose is taken up by the myocardium. The count density of the myocardial images is therefore low, with high background levels. Third, the low energy emission at 80 keV leads to low resolution images with significant attenuation by soft tissues. Technetium-99m (Tc-99m) compounds do not suffer the first and third of these problems and this has encouraged the development of such tracers.

Among the Tc-99m compounds, the most common are Tc-99m-2-methoxy-isobutyl-isonitrile (MIBI) and Tc-99m-1,2-bis[bis(2-ethoxyethyl) phosphino] ethane (Tetrofosmin)[7–9]. In contrast with thallium-201, these two Tc-99m tracers show little redistribution over time, so that separate injections have to be given in order to assess stress and resting perfusion. An important consequence of the lack of significant redistribution of the Tc-99m-labelled agents is that they can be used in the emergency department, catheter laboratory, or in the coronary care unit immediately before thrombolysis. There is ample evidence that resting imaging with Tc-99m-MIBI or Tc-99m-Tetrofosmin is useful in the triage of patients with acute chest pain and non-diagnostic ECGs[10,11]. Recent data suggest that a strategy that incorporates perfusion imaging in such patients is highly cost effective.

Technetium-99m labelled agents may also be used in patients with acute myocardial infarction, not only for diagnostic purposes but to assess the extent of myocardium at risk and determine the effects of therapeutic interventions. In such patients, a Tc-99m-MIBI or Tc-99m-Tetrofosmin injection can be given at the time of presentation in the emergency department, before recanalisation with thrombolytic agents or direct angioplasty. Later reinjection and imaging allow the amount of myocardium that has been salvaged to be established. Another consequence of the lack of redistribution is the ability to perform ventricular function studies either by following the first pass of the tracer through the heart or by electrocardiographically gated acquisition of the myocardial image[12].

Other benefits from the use of Tc-99m agents include the lower radiation burden to patients, and the ability to acquire better quality images in obese patients and women with large breasts. The latter is achievable because Tc-99m provides high photon flux and has short half-life (six hours), which allows higher injected doses. The maximum dose recommended for routine use in the UK is 300 MBq for planar imaging and 400 MBq for tomography, with total doses of 800 MBq and 1000 MBq respectively if stress and rest studies are performed on the same day. 1000 MBq correspond to an effective dose equivalent of 10 mSv.

In clinical practice, the sensitivity of Tc-99m-labelled agents to detect angiographic CAD is similar to that of thallium-201, although some investigators have reported higher values of specificity with Tc-99m-MIBI, particularly when the former is used for investigation of women with chest pain. Both Tc-99 agents have also been used for assessment of hibernating myocardium, but current balance of favour supports thallium-201 as a superior marker of hibernation. In a small number of recent studies, however, sensitivity and specificity values of Tc-99m-MIBI for predicting functional recovery after revascularisation were as high as 100 and 86% respectively, and so it is undeniably a useful radiotracer[13].

3. Are all the perfusion defects due to CAD? Is MPI more specific or sensitive than an exercise test?

Defects of tracer uptake indicate inequalities of tracer delivery to the myocardium or of its active uptake by the myocytes, but this need not always be the result of atheromatous coronary artery disease. Other causes of abnormal scans include coronary artery spasm, anomalous coronary arteries or arteries constricted by muscle bridges, small vessel disease, cardiomyopathies, hypertrophy caused by outflow obstruction or hypertension, infiltrative disorders such as sarcoidosis and amyloidosis, connective tissue disorders and conduction defects such as left bundle branch block[14]. Experienced nuclear cardiologists however, can easily recognise the cause of a perfusion abnormality and typical values of sensitivity and specificity are 95 and 90% respectively. These values are higher than those of an exercise ECG (68 and 77%)[15] but this does not imply that the latter should be replaced by a nuclear study whenever a stress study is required.

Before a decision is made, several variables should be considered and among them, the most important are the radiation burden to the patient, the cost, the comparative risk and benefits of other diagnostic modalities and the pre-test likelihood of CAD in patients being tested. For example, in patients with a low probability of CAD, a stress MPI study as a first line examination is not justified. If patients of this group need a stress study, an exercise ECG is most appropriate and only if it is positive is a myocardial scintigram essential.

4. Why would one request a myocardial perfusion scan?

MPI is the most appropriate diagnostic test for patients with an intermediate probability of CAD. This category includes patients with atypical chest pain, or asymptomatic individuals with a positive exercise ECG, and those with equivocal ST segment changes or a normal exercise ECG despite a history of typical angina. In addition, a myocardial perfusion imaging study should be the first examination when a stress study is required in patients with an uninterpretable exercise ECG because of resting abnormalities (left bundle branch block, pre-excitation, left ventricular hypertrophy, drug effects)[16].

A special case is the asymptomatic patient with risk factors of CAD. Although it is not unreasonable to perform MPI in asymptomatic patients with hypertension or hypercholesterolaemia, it should be emphasised that even in these patients the risk of coronary artery disease is not sufficiently high that the post-test likelihood of disease following an abnormal thallium scan exceeds 50%. This implies that accurate interpretation of such scans is difficult and there is a strong possibility that doctors without good experience in nuclear cardiology will give more false than true positive results in this population. Only in patients with established peripheral vascular disease does the pre-test likelihood of coronary disease reach a sufficiently high level to warrant stress testing in patients without cardiac symptoms. The patient with claudication or an abdominal aortic aneurysm may therefore have an isotope scan (with vasodilators or dobutamine) in order to gauge the risk of vascular surgery[17].

The most valuable contribution that isotope imaging can make to the management of patients (regardless of age or sex) with known or suspected coronary artery disease is to assess the likelihood of a future event such as myocardial infarction and death[18]. Assessment of prognosis helps to guide therapeutic decisions, and these are strongly influenced by the extent and severity of inducible ischaemia which can be objectively assessed by MPI. The latter not only provides the best independent predictors but also gives additional prognostic information of future cardiac events, compared with clinical, exercise electrocardiographic and angiographic data[19].

Perfusion variables that serve as predictors of future events are:

1. The number of transient perfusion defects, which indicate myocardium at risk.
2. The extent of the initial (post stress) defect.
3. The severity of reversibility
4. The nature of the defect (transient, fixed or mixed).

Among the non-perfusion markers, the most important are the amount of post-stress lung uptake of thallium-201 and transient cavity dilatation.

A normal study suggests that the likelihood of a coronary event such as myocardial infarction or death is less than 1% per year, at least over a period of 24 months, a rate close to that of the normal age-matched population[20]. This is independent of the type of imaging agent (thallium-201 or technetium-99m), method of stressing (exercise or pharmacological), population studied (elderly, male or female) and reason for stress testing (patients with known or suspected CAD, after PTCA or CABG). An abnormal study with a small post-stress perfusion defect is also suggestive of a relatively low likelihood of future events (<2% per year), but as the size of the perfusion defect increases so does the likelihood (**Fig. 5.4**).

It could be argued that myocardial perfusion imaging should be performed in all patients with coronary artery disease in order to assess prognosis and to select patients who, irrespective of symptoms, deserve intervention in order to prevent future infarction or death. Such a policy assumes that intervention, even in patients with few or absent symptoms but large areas of inducible ischaemia, can improve prognosis. However, the optimum threshold (amount of myocardium at risk) for which intervention could be beneficial still remains to be determined.

MPI also plays an important role in the management of patients who have suffered an acute myocardial infarction[21]. Patients at intermediate risk by clinical criteria would benefit by direct referral for a stress MPI. The type of stress testing can be either sub-maximal exercise 5 to 7 days after the onset of symptoms, or pharmacological stressing (with vasodilators) as early as 3 to 4 days after admission. A strongly positive scan will identify the high-risk group who will be directed to invasive evaluation, while a scan with small perfusion abnormalities will separate the low-risk patients who will receive medical treatment.

Another group of patients where MPI can accurately assess the prognosis is those with unstable angina. Low- to intermediate-risk in-patients who have been medically stabilised could be stressed safely with either adenosine or dipyridamole within 72 hours of the admission. Using the same prognostic indicators the scan would separate the high- and low-risk sub-groups and determine the future management[22].

Yet another application of MPI is evaluation of patients with chest pain after revascularization. In this group, MPI is useful not only to confirm or rule out the presence of myocardial ischaemia but it can also provide important prognostic information.

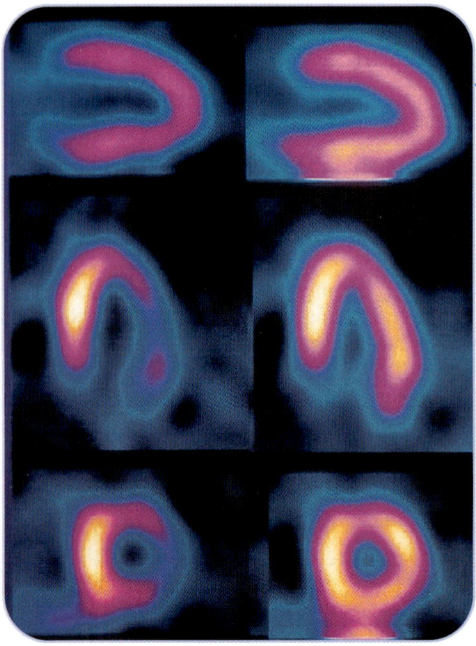

Fig. 5.4
Tomographic stress and rest ^{99m}Tc-tetrofosmin images from a patient with angina. The scan shows inducible ischaemia in most of the myocardium sparing only the septum. The appearances suggest a high likelihood of future cardiac events. Invasive investigation was arranged urgently and a CABG was performed immediately afterwards.

References

1. Verani MS, Mahmarian JJ, Hixson JB, *et al*. Diagnosis of coronary artery disease by controlled coronary vasodilation with adenosine and thallium-201 scintigraphy in patients unable to exercise. *Circulation* 1990;**82**:80.
2. Pennell DJ, Underwood SR, Swanton RH, *et al*.. Dobutamine thallium myocardial perfusion tomography. *J Am Coll Cardiol* 1991;**18**:1471.
3. Weich H, Strauss HW, Pitt B. The extraction of thallium-201 by the myocardium. *Circulation* 1977;**56**:188.
4. Ingwall JS, Kramer M, Kloner NM, *et al*. Thallium accumulation: differentiation between reversible and irreversible myocardial injury. *Circulation* 1979;**59**:678.
5. Dilsizian V, Rocco TP, Freedman NMT, *et al*. Enhanced detection of ischaemic but viable myocardium by the reinjection of thallium after stress-redistribution imaging. *N Engl J Med* 1990;**323**:141.
6. Bax JJ, Wijns W, Cornel JH, *et al*. Accuracy of currently available techniques for prediction of functional recovery after revascularization in patients with left ventricular dysfunction due to chronic coronary artery disease; Comparison of pooled data. *J Am Coll Cardiol* 1997;**30**:1451.
7. Heo J, Kegel J, Iskandrian AS, *et al*. Comparison of same-day protocols using technetium-99m-sestamibi myocardial imaging. *J Nucl Med* 1992;**33**:186.
8. Taillefer R. Technetium-99m sestamibi myocardial imaging: same-day rest-stress studies and dipyridamole. *Am J Cardiol* 1990;**66**:80.
9. Sridhara B, Sochor H, Rigo P, *et al*. Myocardial single-photon emission computed tomographic imaging with technetium 99m tetrofosmin: stress-rest imaging with same-day and separate-day rest imaging. *J Nucl Cardiol* 1994;**2(1)**:138.
10. Kontos MC, Jesse RL, Schmidt KL, *et al*. Value of acute rest sestamibi perfusion imaging for evaluation of patients admitted to the emergency department with chest pain. *J Am Coll Cardiol* 1997;**30(4)**:976.
11. Heller GV, Stowers SA, Hendel RC, *et al*. Clinical value of acute rest technetium-99m tetrofosmin tomographic myocardial perfusion imaging in patients with acute chest pain and nondiagnostic electrocardiograms. *J Am Coll Cardiol* 1998;**31**:1011.
12. Anagnostopoulos C, Gunning MG, Pennell DJ, *et al*.. Regional myocardial motion and thickening assessed by ECG-Gated ^{99m}Tc-MIBI emission tomography and by magnetic resonance imaging. *Eur J Nucl Med* 1996;**23**:909.
13. Maublant JC, Citron B, Lipiecki J, *et al*. Rest technetium-99m sestamibi scintigraphy in hibernating myocardium. *Am Heart J* 1995;**129**:306.
14. Braat SH, Brugada P, Bar FW, *et al*. Thallium-201 exercise scintigraphy and left bundle branch block. *Am J Cardiol* 1985;**55**:224.
15. Gianrossi R, Detrano R, Mulvihill D, *et al*. Exercise induced ST depression in the diagnosis of coronary artery disease: a meta-analysis. *Circulation* 1989:**80**:87.
16. De Bono D, for the Joint Working Party of the British Cardiac Society and Royal of Physicians of London. Investigation and management of stable angina: revised guidelines 1998. *Heart* 1999;**81**:546.
17. Leppo J, Plaja J, Gionet M, *et al*. Noninvasive evaluation of cardiac risk before elective vascular surgery. *J Am Coll Cardiol* 1987;**9**:269.
18. Ladenheim ML, Kotler TS, Pollock BH, *et al*. Incremental prognostic power of clinical history, exercise electrocardiography and myocardial perfusion scintigraphy in suspected coronary artery disease. *Am J Cardiol* 1987;**59**:270.
19. Marie PY, Danchin N, Durand JF, *et al*. Long-term prediction of major ischemic events by exercise thallium-201 single-photon emission computed tomography. Incremental prognostic value compared with clinical, exercise testing, catheterization and radionuclide angiographic data. *J Am Coll Cardiol* 1995;**26(4)**:879.
20. Iskander S, Iskandrian AE. Risk assessment using single-photon emission computed tomographic technetium-99m sestamibi imaging. *J Am Coll Cardiol* 1998;**32**:57.
21. Berman D, Hachamovitch R, Lewin H, *et al*. Risk stratification in coronary artery disease: implications for stabilization and prevention. *Am J Cardiol* 1997;**79(12B)**:10.
22. Miller DD, Stratmann HG, Shaw L, *et al*. Dipyridamole technetium 99m sestamibi myocardial tomography as an independent predictor of cardiac event-free survival after acute ischemic events. *J Nucl Cardiol* 1994;**1**:72.

6. Cardiovascular Magnetic Resonance in the Diagnosis and Management of Angina

Nick Bellenger
Dudley Pennell

1. What is cardiovascular magnetic resonance (CMR)?

Magnetic resonance uses magnetic fields and radiowaves to generate high resolution images. CMR uses this technology, together with a combination of fast sequences, ECG gating and respiratory tracking to obtain static and cine images of the heart that are free of motion artefact.

2. What can CMR do?

CMR is the reference standard for structural abnormalities of the heart and great vessels, and is routinely used in the diagnosis of congenital and valvular heart disease. The high reproducibility also allows for accurate temporal assessment of progressive disorders such as aortic dissection and heart failure. Non-invasive assessment of both global and regional function, tissue characterisation, myocardial perfusion and coronary angiography are all possible by CMR. Additional techniques such quantification of blood flow velocity and contrast angiography augment the versatility of this rapidly expanding imaging modality.

3. What are the advantages of CMR over alternative imaging techniques?

CMR can generate static or cine images of higher spatial and temporal resolution than other techniques. These images are not limited by the attenuation artefacts of nuclear cardiology, or by the limitations of acoustic windows of echocardiography. Furthermore, CMR images can be acquired in any desired plane without exposure to contrast agents or ionising radiation.

4. How can CMR be used in the assessment of angina?

CMR can provide information on ischaemic heart disease through the assessment of rest and stress wall motion, myocardial perfusion and coronary artery anatomy.

5. How does CMR measure wall motion?

The ability to generate cine images with high temporal resolution allows a qualitative assessment of regional cardiac function similar to echocardiography. However, there are no acoustic window limitations. CMR can provide images in any plane but the vertical long axis, horizontal long axis (**Fig. 6.1**) and a stack of contiguous short axis cine slices encompassing the whole of the left and right ventricle are usually used (**Fig. 6.2**). These views ensure that every myocardial segment is examined in detail[1,2]. These views can be reproduced accurately for follow-up or rest–stress studies. A further advantage of CMR is the potential for quantitative wall motion assessment. Although a number of methods are available, this is best achieved by a process called tagging[3] where a non-invasive imaging grid is superimposed on the myocardium, allowing direct analysis of the three-dimensional distortion of the myocardium (**Fig. 6.3**). Tagging is achieved by laying down the grid of lines of magnetic saturation at end-diastole. These distort as the heart contracts, and the change in the intersection points of the grid can be followed by cine imaging. These images are then subjected to a quantitative computer analysis to generate myocardial strain and other contraction variables. Myocardial dynamics are more complicated than simple wall thickening, and two-dimensional motion and tagging allows assessment of the complex interaction of contraction, expansion, twisting and through plane motion[4].

6. Can cardiac stress testing be performed in the magnet?

CMR can be used to assess stress-induced ischaemic wall motion abnormality and identify reversible ischaemia in the same way as echocardiography The use of exercise has been reported, but the physical constraints of the magnet make it difficult. Thus, pharmacological stress agents are generally used[5,6].

7. How does stress MR compare with stress echocardiography?

Low dose dobutamine CMR has been shown to be comparable with stress echocardiography[7] and positron emission tomography[1] for detecting viable myocardium, while high dose dobutamine CMR has been shown to have superior sensitivity and specificity for the detection of coronary artery disease[8]. This is because CMR is considerably more accurate in patients in whom stress echocardiography is limited by suboptimal imaging.

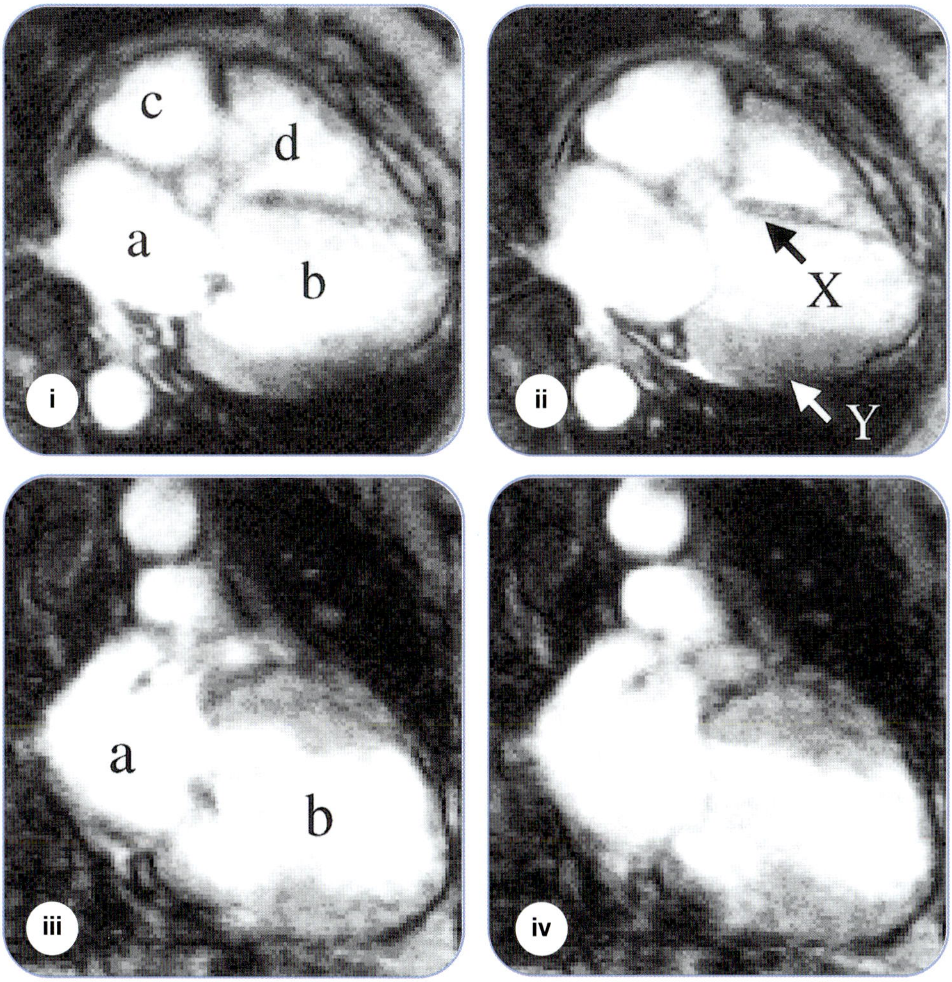

Fig. 6.1 CMR in the horizontal long axis (HLA) (i and ii), and vertical long axis (VLA) (iii and iv) in both diastole (i and iii) and systole (ii and iv). Each image represents one frame out of a 16 frame cine. This patient has suffered an antero-septal myocardial infarction and demonstrates thinning of the myocardium, poor wall motion and absent myocardial thickening in this region (X). In comparison, the lateral wall shows good contraction and thickening (Y). a, left atrium; b, left ventricle; c, right atrium; d, right ventricle.

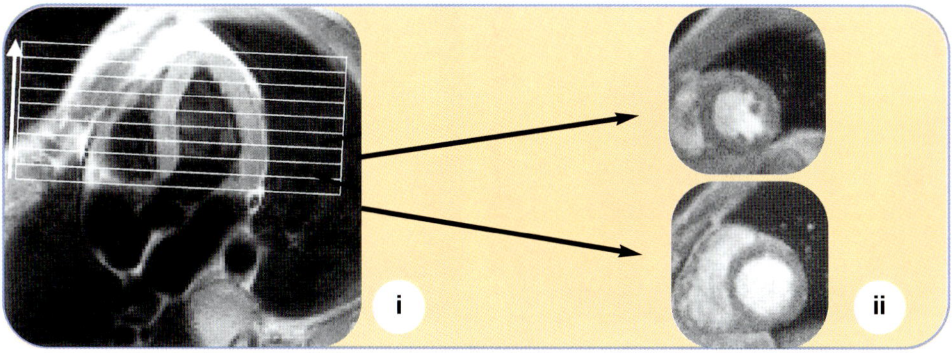

Fig. 6.2 A stack of (in this case 9) short axis (SA) images (ii) are acquired from the HLA (i). Each SA slice is 10 mm thick and consists of a multi-frame cine. Each myocardial segment can be assessed for wall motion.

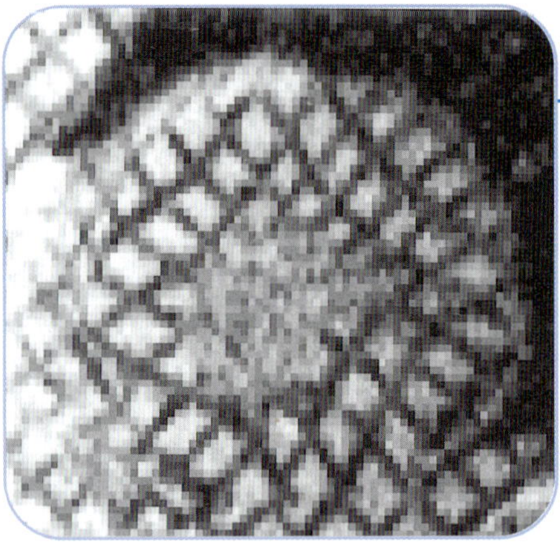

Fig. 6.3
An SA slice with myocardial tagging lines present. These lines remain in place over the cardiac cycle and become distorted as regional contraction, expansion and twisting occurs. Courtesy of C Kramer, Allegheny General Hospital, Pittsburgh, USA.

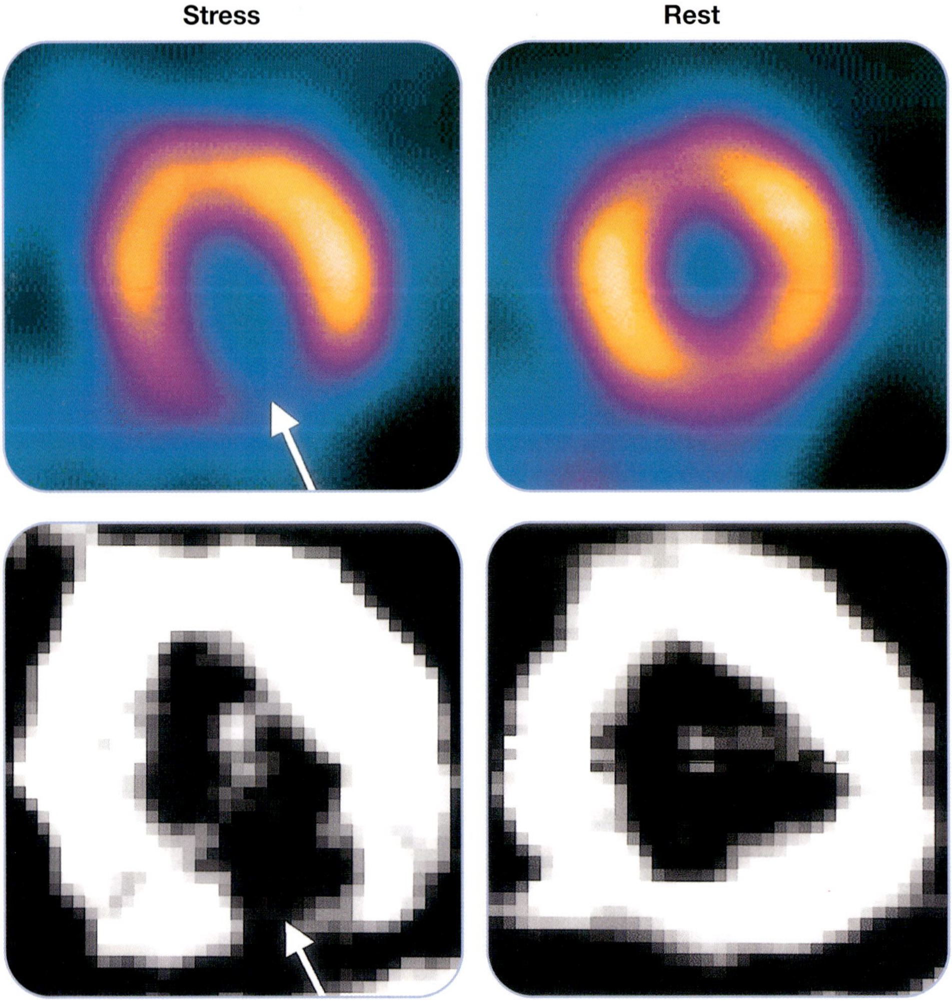

Fig. 6.4 An example of a reversible inferior defect (arrow) by single slice EPI CMR perfusion compared with thallium SPECT. Courtesy of J Panting, CMR Unit, Royal Brompton Hospital, London, UK.

8. How does CMR measure myocardial perfusion?

CMR can assess myocardial perfusion by utilising ultrafast imaging sequences with multiple slices of the heart acquired at every heart beat during the first pass of a paramagnetic contrast agent. Myocardium perfused by a diseased vessel shows a lower peak signal intensity, a lower rate of signal increase and a longer time to peak than myocardium perfused by normal vessels (**Fig. 6.4**). Parametric maps of perfusion can be generated, closely resembling the results from nuclear cardiology techniques.

9. How does CMR perfusion compare with other techniques?

CMR perfusion imaging correlates well with vasodilator thallium scintigraphy and coronary angiography[9,10]. Scintigraphy, however, is limited by lower spatial resolution and also requires exposure to radiation. CMR allows more accurate definition of perfusion defects, including the ability to differentiate sub-endocardial defects. Newer CMR contrast agents also hold promise for providing quantitative measures of perfusion[11].

10. Can CMR image coronary arteries?

As a result of significant technical advances, the problems of the effects of cardiac and respiratory motion on imaging such small vessels as the coronaries have now been largely overcome. This, together with improved spatial resolution, has led to wider use of CMR to image coronary arteries (**Fig. 6.5**). CMR has established its value in the assessment of anomalous coronary arteries, where it has been shown to be superior to angiography[12], as well as coronary artery bypass grafts[13]. Stenoses in native vessels can be detected with reasonable sensitivity and specificity[14], but this is not in common use, while measurement of coronary flow velocity holds promise for the future[15]. CMR has been used in patients in whom X-ray coronary angiography has proved problematic[16], and also to define whether the infarct related artery is patent after myocardial infarction[17].

11. What is the patient required to do?

Patients are required to lie on a couch that moves within the bore of a magnet. Claustrophobic patients may find this difficult, but sedation can be safely administered if necessary. Once inside, the patient will not feel anything but will notice some background noise as the images are acquired.

12. Is it safe?

There are no known hazards associated with the exposure to radio frequency or high-intensity magnetic fields. Care must be taken not to use any non-MR-compatible equipment in the vicinity of the magnetic field, including routine crash trolley equipment, to prevent any possibility of ferromagnetic objects being attracted into the bore of the magnet.

In the acute setting or for stress studies, CMR compatible equipment can now provide monitoring of all the routine haemodynamic parameters including those obtained from invasive methods. MR-compatible ventilators and shorter scanners that allow better access to the patient have been developed to allow scanning in the acute situation[18].

13. Are there any contraindications?

Contraindications include implantable devices such as defibrillators, cochlear implants or cerebral aneurysm clips. Patients with pacemakers should not be scanned, although some specialised approaches are available, in expert cardiac centres only, for patients with an overwhelming clinical case for MR scanning. A wide range of prostheses

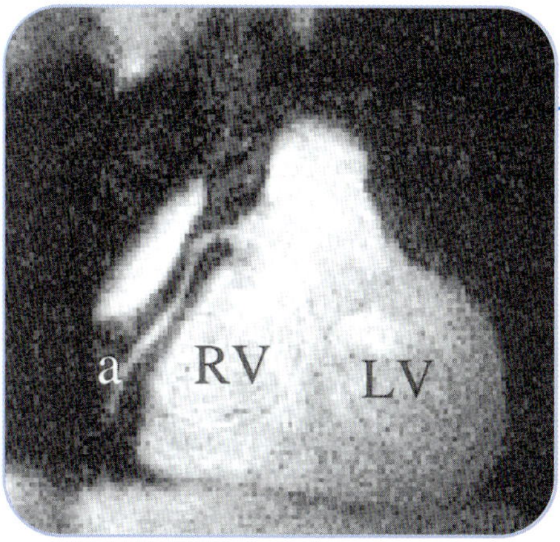

Fig. 6.5
Right coronary artery (a) by spiral CMR. This image was acquired non-invasively without the use of a contrast agent or ionizing radiation. RV, right ventricle; LV, left ventricle. Courtesy of A Taylor, CMR Unit, Royal Brompton Hospital, London, UK.

are now MR-compatible and do not prevent scanning, including prosthetic heart valves and intra-coronary stents. Sternal wires will cause a localised loss of signal, although these are usually located anterior to the heart and rarely interfere with the images.

14. Is CMR generally available now?

At present, CMR is available in only a few specialised centres in the UK, but use of the technique is expanding rapidly and it should become more widely available.

15. What can be requested now?

This depends on the centre, but routine assessments include anatomical and structural abnormalities as well as assessment of left and right cardiac volumes, mass and function. Qualitative wall motion analysis is easily performed but quantitative assessment, myocardial perfusion and coronary artery pathology is often restricted to more specialised units. Both industry and medicine are experiencing a rapid growth in CMR technology, availability, knowledge and experience so it is unlikely to be long before CMR referrals are commonplace for junior doctors.

References

1. Matheijssen NA, De Roos A, Doornbos J, *et al.* Left ventricular wall motion analysis in patients with acute myocardial infarction using magnetic resonance imaging. *Magn Reson Imaging* 1993;**11(4)**:485–92.
2. Bellenger NG, Francis JM, Davies LC, *et al.* Establishment and performance of a magnetic resonance cardiac function clinic. *J Cardiovasc Magn Reson* 2000;**2**:15–18.
3. Geskin G, Kramer CM, Rogers WJ, *et al.*. Quantitative assessment of myocardial viability after infarction by dobutamine magnetic resonance tagging. *Circulation* 1998;**98**:217–3.
4. Zerhouni EA, Parish DM, Rogers WJ, *et al.* Human heart: tagging with MR imaging – a method for noninvasive assessment of myocardial motion. *Radiology* 1988;**169(1)**:59–63.
5. Pennell DL, Underwood SR, Manzara CC, *et al.* Magnetic resonance imaging during dobutamine stress in coronary artery disease. *Am J Cardiol* 1992;**70(1)**:34–40.
6. Nagel E, Lehmkuhl H, Vogel U, *et al.* High dose dobutamine stress magnetic resonance tomography for the non-invasive detection of wall motion abnormalities. *Circulation* 1999; **99**:763–70.
7. Dendale PA, Franken PR, Waldman GJ, *et al.*. Low-dosage dobutamine magnetic resonance imaging as an alternative to echocardiography in the detection of viable myocardium after acute infarction. *Am Heart J* 1995;**130(1)**:134–40.
8. Baer FM, Voth E, Schneider CA, *et al.* Comparison of low-dose dobutamine-gradient-echo magnetic resonance imaging and positron emission tomography with [18F]fluorodeoxyglucose in patients with chronic coronary artery disease. A functional and morphological approach to the detection of residual myocardial viability. *Circulation* 1995;**91**:1006–15.
9. Kivellitz DE, Wilke NM, Bis KG, *et al.* Quantitative MR first pass versus N13-ammonia PET perfusion imaging in coronary artery disease. *Radiology* 1997;**205(Suppl.)**:253.
10. Schaefer S, van Tyen R, Saloner D. Evaluation of myocardial perfusion abnormalities with gadolinium enhanced snapshot MR imaging in humans. *Radiology* 1992;**185**:795–801.
11. Taylor AM, Panting JR, Keegan J, *et al.* Use of the intravascular contrast agent NC100150 injection in spin echo and gradient echo imaging of the heart. *J Cardiovasc Magn Reson* 1999;**1**:23–32.
12. Post JC, Van Rossum AC, Hofman MBM, *et al.* Clinical utility of two-dimensional magnetic resonance angiography in detecting coronary artery disease. *Eur Heart J* 1997;**18**:426–33.
13. Galjee MA, Van Rossum AC, Doesburg T, *et al.* Value of magnetic resonance imaging in assessing patency and function of coronary artery bypass grafts. *Circulation* 1996;**93**:660–6.
14. Pennell DJ, Bogren HG, Keegan J, *et al.* Assessment of coronary artery stenosis by magnetic resonance imaging. *Heart* 1996;**75(2)**:127–33.
15. Keegan J, Firmin D, Gatehouse P, *et al.* The application of breath-hold phase velocity mapping techniques to the measurement of coronary artery blood flow velocity: Phantom data and initial in vivo results. *Magn Reson Med* 1994;**31**:526–36.
16. Warner OJ, Ohri SK, Pennell DJ, *et al.* Magnetic resonance coronary artery imaging for redo cardiac surgery. *Ann Thorac Surg* 1996:**62**:1513–16.
17. Hundley WG, Clarke GD, Lansau C, *et al.* Noninvasive determination of infarct artery patency by cine magnetic resonance angiography. *Circulation* 1995;**91**:1347–53.
18. Bellenger N, Pennell DJ. Magnetic resonance imaging: A role in ITU? *Int J Intensive Care* 1999;**9(Suppl)**:43-50

7. Coronary Angiography in the Management of Angina

Miles Dalby

1. What are the indications for coronary angiography?

As with any invasive test in medicine, the decision of whether or not to undertake coronary angiography should take account of the balance between the risk to the patient and the likely benefits. Decisions about cardiac catheterisation, therefore, need to be taken in the context of the individual patient and no set of guidelines can replace this. Furthermore, although registry data is available, there is little prospective trial-based evidence for practice with regard to diagnostic procedures. The following however provides a framework which may help guide clinical practice.

The indications for coronary angiography can be categorised according to the clinical presentation. Enthusiasm for cardiac catheterisation varies between individual clinicians, and between countries both because of clinical opinion and available resource. Much of this review is based on the American Heart Association/American College of Cardiology guidelines for coronary angiography, published in May 1999[1,2], with information from the British Cardiac Society/Royal College of Physicians working-party guidelines on the investigation and management of stable angina, also published in May 1999[3].

Chest pain suspicious of coronary artery disease or in the presence of known coronary artery disease

In the former context, coronary angiography allows confirmation of coronary artery disease (CAD) in addition to assessment of severity of disease. Known CAD implies documentary objective evidence, which means prior coronary angiography or confirmed myocardial infarction. In such patients, the presence of coronary disease is not in doubt. The purpose of the test is to stratify risk and to assess the potential for revascularisation, be it surgical or percutaneous. Generally agreed indications for angiography in these clinical contexts include:

1. Severe angina refractory to medical treatment.
2. High-risk criteria on non-invasive testing.
3. Patients resuscitated from 'sudden cardiac death'.
4. Sustained ventricular tachycardia.

There is debate regarding the following indications, in which the individual patient, available resources and physician preference will guide investigations:

1. Less severe angina or that which responds well to medical therapy.
2. Documented but non-high-risk patterns of ischaemia on non-invasive testing.
3. Patients in whom non-invasive testing is difficult to perform or interpret. In this case the decision will largely be based on the clinical history and the presence of risk factors.
4. Previous myocardial infarction, with normal left ventricular function and the absence of high risk criteria on non-invasive testing.

There is general agreement that coronary angiography is not indicated in the following circumstances:

1. Angina in patients who are not candidates for revascularisation.
2. Angina in patients who do not wish to undergo revascularisation, even if indicated.

Unstable angina

Unstable angina is a clinical syndrome which carries a very high morbidity and mortality, and as such should be investigated and treated as a matter of urgency. Generally agreed indications for angiography in this clinical context include:

1. Clinically high-risk unstable angina (prolonged pain, pain not responding to treatment, ECG changes).
2. Unstable angina with a clinically low-risk presentation but subsequent high-risk findings on non-invasive testing.

There is debate regarding the role of coronary angiography in unstable angina in the context of clinical low-risk presentation with subsequent lack of high risk criteria on non-invasive testing.

Although patients with 'high-risk' unstable angina tend to undergo early or emergency angiography in clinical practice, the place of early *interventional* management in the clinical context of acute coronary syndromes is unclear and this matter is the subject of contemporary clinical trials.

Non-specific chest pain

In general, such patients should undergo angiography only in the presence of high-risk findings on non-invasive testing. It should generally be avoided in patients with normal findings on non-invasive investigation. It may be necessary, however, to perform angiography in such patients who are recurrently admitted to hospital with chest pain, and although there is little evidence to support it, a normal angiogram may be reassuring to both patient and physician.

Other specific scenarios

There are a number of other clinical scenarios which do not fit well into the above classification. These include acute myocardial infarction, in which early angiography and interventional management may be beneficial, and possibly superior to, thrombolysis, but are beyond the scope of this review.

2. Is cardiac catheterisation the gold standard in diagnosis and how much information is gathered during the examination?

Over recent years, remarkable advances have been made in the non-invasive assessment of CAD. In addition to the traditional treadmill exercise test, which remains an extremely useful investigation, myocardial perfusion imaging, magnetic resonance imaging (MRI) and computerised axial tomography (CAT) are increasingly used. Such tests can allow low-risk cases to be managed without angiography, and allow expeditious angiography in high-risk cases. This removes the risk of the procedure to the very low-risk patient, and allows health care resources to be directed to higher risk patients.

Furthermore, although coronary angiography gives a detailed anatomical record of the coronary arteries and their stenoses, there is a limit to what it can offer since it only delineates the lumen of the artery. Its shortcomings are well summarised in the BCS/RCP guidelines:

> *"Strictly speaking it does not... diagnose either coronary atheroma (since vessel wall disease may be present when the lumen is normal) or myocardial ischaemia (since it does not give full information about coronary flow)".*

However, in contemporary practice, coronary angiography:

- remains the only modality available for detailed and full anatomical assessment of the coronary arteries;
- allows risk stratification; and
- is mandatory for assessment of the feasibility, need for and method of revascularisation.

Although the principal aim of the investigation is to define the coronary artery anatomy, a great deal of further information can be gained. It also allows a left ventricular angiogram to be performed to assess LV dimensions, overall function and look for the presence of any regional wall motion abnormalities. Aortic valve stenosis can be assessed by measuring the pressure gradient between LV and aorta. Aortic and mitral valve regurgitation can be qualitatively assessed by visualisation of regurgitant dye. Finally, if a venous catheter is passed into the right heart, further information, including cardiac output and pulmonary and systemic haemodynamic data, can be gained.

Thus although other tests may reduce the need for angiography in some low-risk clinical situations, in contemporary practice the test remains the gold standard, and it is mandatory if revascularisation is being considered.

3. What risks are involved?

As with all invasive tests in medicine, there are risks involved. The mortality and morbidity of the examination depend on the individual case. The overall mortality in the American report of the Registry of the Society of Cardiac Angiography and Intervention (SCA&I) in 1991 was 0.11%[4]. The UK registry experience indicated a remarkably similar overall mortality of 0.12% in 1993[5]. Two much smaller single-centre reports from the west of England in 1999 have reported mortalities of 0.07 and 0.01%[6,7]. Patients with an increased mortality rate include those with hypertension, shock, renal insufficiency, unstable angina, significant LAD disease, poor left ventricular function, aortic valve disease, mitral valve disease, myocardial infarction within 24 hours, cardiomyopathy, three-vessel coronary artery disease and advanced age. In one series, cardiac catheterisation in patients over the age of 80 years gave a mortality of nearly 1%[8].

The 1993 UK registry data indicated an overall risk of a serious complications of 0.8%, with an emergency surgical intervention rate of 0.08%. The risk of a cerebrovascular event causing death or permanent neurological damage was 0.02%. Reactions to angiographic contrast are common, particularly with ionic agents. Although these are usually minor, ventricular arrhythmias are sometimes induced, particularly when imaging grafts, or during accidental injection of the conus branch of the right coronary artery. With electrical cardioversion facilities immediately available, these complications rarely lead to significant morbidity or mortality. It is also rare for contrast medium-induced bradycardia to cause significant long-term effects.

Using the femoral approach, vascular complications include arterial occlusion, retroperitoneal bleeding, haematoma, false aneurysm, arteriovenous fistula formation and infection. The risk of requiring surgical repair of false aneurysm, however, is low, and digital pressure or pressure over the neck of the aneurysm with an ultrasound probe will often resolve the situation. Rates of femoral vascular access complications actually requiring surgical intervention are very low and in the single centre report from Exeter the rate was 0.17%[6].

Most series suggest that the risk of access site complications is higher when the brachial approach is used, and the Exeter study found a rate of 0.24%. Unfavourable experience with this route, however, may relate to the experience of operators. The American CASS study found that angiography using the brachial route resulted in over three times the mortality with the femoral route except in centres with 80% or more brachial procedures[9].

4. When would brachial rather than groin access be undertaken?

Cardiac catheterisation via the brachial artery has benefits in certain clinical situations, including:

- Patients receiving anticoagulation which cannot be stopped, or patients in whom the international normalised ratio (INR) remains high, having stopped it shortly before the procedure.

- Significant femoral artery atheroma or vascular surgery, where access from the leg may be difficult, or may result in distal embolisation.
- Aortic stenosis, where it may be easier to cross the stenotic valve from the arm than the leg.

Because of the higher potential for access site complications, however, this approach should only be performed by, or under the close supervision of, experienced brachial operators.

5. What is the radiation burden to the patient?

Calculation of the radiation dose during diagnostic coronary angiography is complex. Two intensities of radiation are used: that for screening while manipulating and engaging catheters, and that for acquiring when actually recording images for subsequent viewing. Different laboratories use different equipment; furthermore, screening times differ between patients, and between operators. The UK National Radiological Protection Board recognises this, and in the summary of an advisory group meeting, accepts that although data should be collected so that guidelines can be agreed in the future, it is *"difficult to give achievable doses for angiographic procedures…due to the complexity of the techniques"*[10]. The study from the Newcastle Regional Medical Physics Department in the UK gives data based on over 2000 patients in a single centre. The dose equivalent ranged approximately from 5 to 10 mSv[11]. To express this in terms of actual risk is even more difficult, but assuming a risk of fatal cancer of 5%/Sv and an effective dose of 10 mSv, the average risk per procedure would be about 0.05%. For other ways of expressing this difficult concept, helpful advice on this and related matters is provided in the NRPB website at www.nrpb.org.uk.

While radiation burden is always a concern, coronary angiography is an extremely useful test and the overall risk from a single diagnostic examination is very low.

References

1. Scanlon PJ, Faxon DP, Audet AM, *et al.* ACC/AHA guidelines for coronary angiography: executive summary and recommendations. A report of the American College of Cardiology/American Heart Association Task Force on Practice Guidelines (Committee on Coronary Angiography). Developed in collaboration with the Society for Cardiac Angiography and Interventions. *Circulation* 1999;**99**:2345–57.
2. Scanlon PJ, Faxon DP, Audet AM, *et al.* ACC/AHA guidelines for coronary angiography. A report of the American College of Cardiology/American Heart Association Task Force on Practice Guidelines (Committee on Coronary Angiography). Developed in collaboration with the Society for Cardiac Angiography and Interventions. *J Am Coll Cardiol* 1999;**33**:1756–824.
3. de Bono D. Investigation and management of stable angina: revised guidelines 1998. Joint Working Party of the British Cardiac Society and Royal College of Physicians of London. *Heart* 1999;**81**:546–55.
4. Noto TJJ, Johnson LW, Krone R, *et al.* Cardiac catheterization 1990: a report of the Registry of the Society for Cardiac Angiography and Interventions (SCA&I). *Catheter Cardiovasc Diagn* 1991;**24**:75–83.
5. de Bono D. Complications of diagnostic cardiac catheterisation: results from 34,041 patients in the United Kingdom confidential enquiry into cardiac catheter complications. The Joint Audit Committee of the British Cardiac Society and Royal College of Physicians of London. *Br Heart J* 1993;**70**:297–300.
6. Smith LD, Spyer G, Dean JW. Audit of cardiac catheterisation in a district general hospital: implications for training. *Heart* 1999;**81**:461–4.
7. Papaconstantinou HD, Marshall AJ, Burrell CJ. Diagnostic cardiac catheterisation in a hospital without on-site cardiac surgery. *Heart* 1999;**81**:465–9.
8. Clark VL, Khaja F: Risk of cardiac catheterization in patients aged ≥80 years without previous cardiac surgery. *Am J Cardiol* 1994;**74**:1076–7.
9. Davis K, Kennedy JW, Kemp HGJ, *et al.* Complications of coronary arteriography from the Collaborative Study of Coronary Artery Surgery (CASS). *Circulation* 1979;**59**:1105–12.
10. NRPB. Guidelines on patient dose to promote the optimisation of protection for diagnostic medical exposure. Recommendations 148 and 149. *NRPB* 1999; **10(1)**: 36–40.
11. Broadhead DA, Chapple CL, Faulkner K, *et al.* The impact of cardiology on the collective effective dose in the North of England. *Br J Radiol* 1997;**70**:492–7

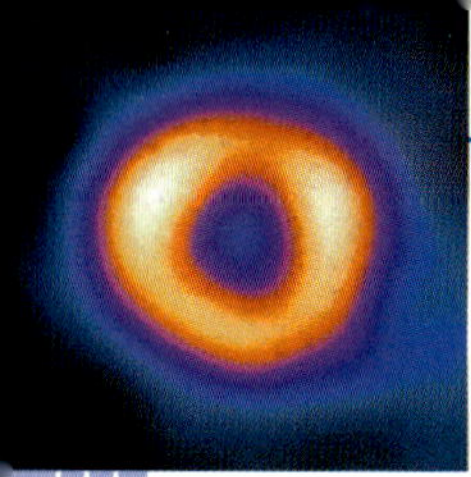

II. Cardiac Symptoms and Pathophysiology

8. Atherosclerosis and Myocardial Ischaemia

Henry Purcell
Sam Kaddoura

1. What is atherosclerosis and what are its effects?

Atherosclerosis is an intimal disease of arteries involving connective tissue proliferation and lipid accumulation. Endothelial dysfunction is central to the pathogenesis of atherosclerosis. The process occurs in focal areas of the intima and is not diffuse[1]. A range of arteries are affected from the aorta downwards to vessels of approximately 3 mm external diameter. Some arteries such as the internal mammary (used widely in bypass graft surgery) are relatively spared, while others such as the coronary arteries are at high risk.

The process of atherosclerosis begins in childhood and progresses slowly over a course of years. The clinical expression of CHD falls into two groups, chronic stable angina and acute syndromes which encompass unstable angina, myocardial infarction and sudden cardiac death. The biological (inflammatory) state of lesions is clearly important in determining the clinical outcome of patients with coronary atherosclerosis[2] and may to a large degree differentiate between chronic stable (static) and acute lesions where plaque disruption and rupture leads to thrombosis with partial or complete occlusion of the artery (**Fig. 8.1**). Most patients with stable angina have one or more areas of high grade stenosis caused by the intimal lesions of atheroma, which reduce the luminal diameter by more than 50%, and have the potential to vary the degree of obstruction as the vasomotor tone changes. These plaques may be eccentric or concentric in shape. The latter, which surround the entire circumference, are more angiographically visible. They may be composed mainly of collagen or lipid. High grade lesions (>70% by diameter) tend to be predominantly collagen.

2. What is the link between angina and atherosclerosis?

The important link between coronary atherosclerosis and angina pectoris was established in the early 1900s. It later became apparent that angina does not necessarily occur as a consequence of failure of coronary blood flow to increase in response to an augmented demand. More recently it was proposed that impaired endothelial vasodilator function might be an important mechanism of myocardial ischaemia. However, there is now evidence that localised chronic inflammatory processes within the atherosclerotic plaque rather than endothelium are responsible not only for plaque rupture but also for the hyperreactivity of these vessels to vasoconstrictor stimuli[3]. While research on the mechanisms of angina continues there is increased interest in the metabolic consequences of myocardial ischaemia and how to afford 'cytoprotection'.

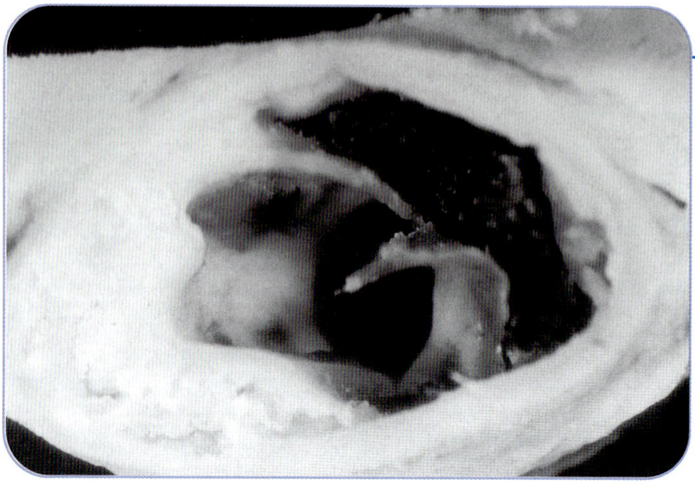

Fig. 8.1
Perfused, fixed human coronary artery showing major plaque rupture with broken fibrous cap flap and intraplaque haemorrhage. Site to the left of lumen shows a further cholesterol-rich plaque. Courtesy of Dr Mary Sheppard.

3. How does myocardial ischaemia occur?

Although conceptually appealing, there are limitations to the traditional definition of myocardial ischaemia, i.e. an imbalance between oxygen supply and demand, since both entities are difficult to measure. A more precise definition has been proposed, whereby ischaemia is characterised by an imbalance of adenosine triphospate (ATP) consumption and blood flow, and the flow-related accumulation of lactic acid[4].

For the heart to pump efficiently it requires vast amounts of energy. It can use a variety of substrates as energy sources but most of its energy is via oxidative metabolism of fatty acids and glucose to form ATP (**Fig. 8.2**)[5]. Fatty acids are oxidised in preference to glucose, but insulin will favour glucose consumption. ATP can be produced anaerobically, though less efficiently by glycolysis. Following coronary occlusion, the glycolytic pathway is stimulated, but ATP and the energy storage form of phosphate, creatine phosphate (CP) (which appears to act as a back-up system providing immediate energy for contraction), become depleted within minutes. As there is inadequate oxygen to allow oxidative phosphorylation, pyruvate (the end product of the glycolytic chain), instead of passing into the citric acid cycle is converted to lactate, which stimulates pain receptors.

Ventricular function in the ischaemic area becomes impaired within a few seconds following coronary occlusion, but is completely reversible if flow is restored promptly. If ischaemia is reversed within 10–15 minutes, the biochemical changes described and myocardial function are fully reversible but it may take several hours for contractility to return fully to normal. If ischaemia is prolonged, however, irreversible damage occurs despite restoration of myocardial perfusion[6].

Sigwart and colleagues were among the first to demonstrate the sequence of events during myocardial ischaemia (**Fig. 8.3**)[7]. They monitored changes during balloon obstruction of the coronary artery in humans. This shows that ischaemia is characterised by a transition period during which it remains silent. Following balloon occlusion there are haemodynamic abnormalities which are followed by electrocardiographic changes before the appearance of painful symptoms.

4. What is the significance of 'silent myocardial ischaemia'?

There has been considerable interest in the clinical phenomenon of silent myocardial ischaemia, as approximately 70% of ischaemic episodes in patients with symptomatic coronary artery disease are not associated with angina[8].

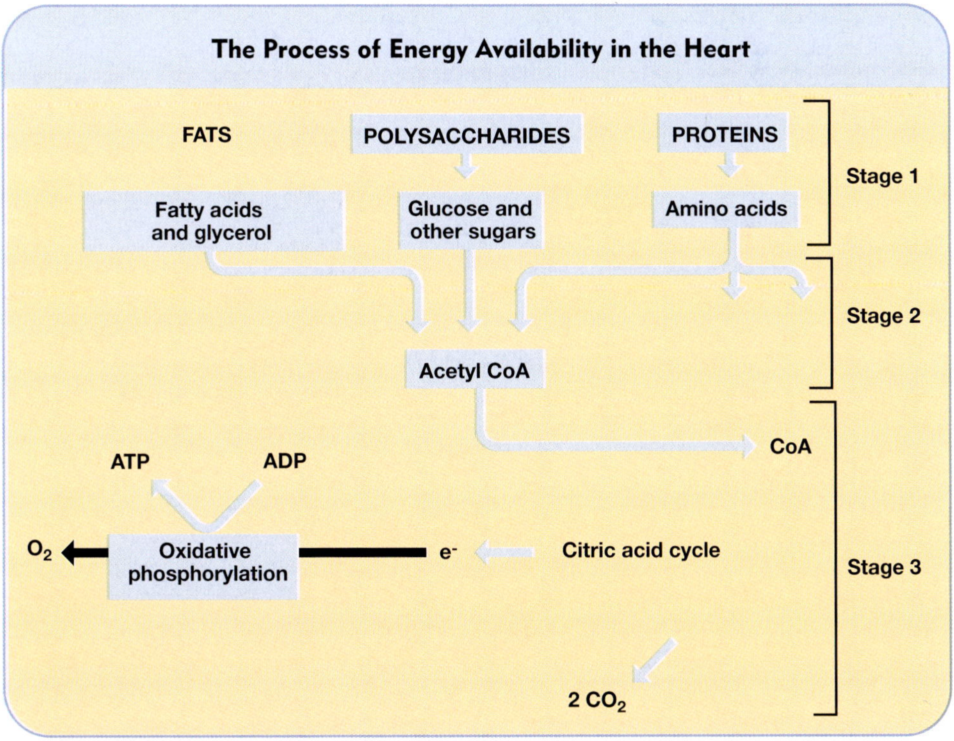

Fig. 8.2 The process of energy availability in the heart. Stage I involves hydrolysis to simple molecules, which are converted (stage 2) into the acetyl unit of acetyl CoA with some generation of ATP, and the final common pathways in the oxidation of energy molecules (stage 3), with ATP produced during oxidative phosphorylation. Reproduced with permission by WH Freeman and Co[5].

Silent ischaemia provides important prognostic information in patients with unstable angina or following acute myocardial infarction (MI). In patients with stable angina, the situation is less clear cut. However, patients in whom exercise-induced ischaemia is silent have a similar prevalence of left main and three-vessel coronary disease and have no lower mortality over subsequent years as compared to those in whom ischaemia is associated with angina.

5. What is the difference between myocardial 'stunning' and 'hibernation'?

The concept of myocardial ischaemia has expanded to embrace the phenomenona of myocardial stunning and hibernation. These terms are used to describe, respectively, a state of prolonged post-ischaemic myocardial dysfunction following severe transient ischaemia, and reduced myocardial inotropy due to a persistent state of reduced coronary blood flow, i.e. chronic ischaemia (**Fig. 8.4**). The difference between them is that 'stunning' represents temporary post-ischaemic dysfunction of the myocardium occurring at a time when coronary blood flow is apparently normal or supranormal. The mechanical dysfunction persists after reperfusion despite the absence of irreversible damage and restoration of normal blood flow. 'Hibernation', by contrast, is a condition of reduced

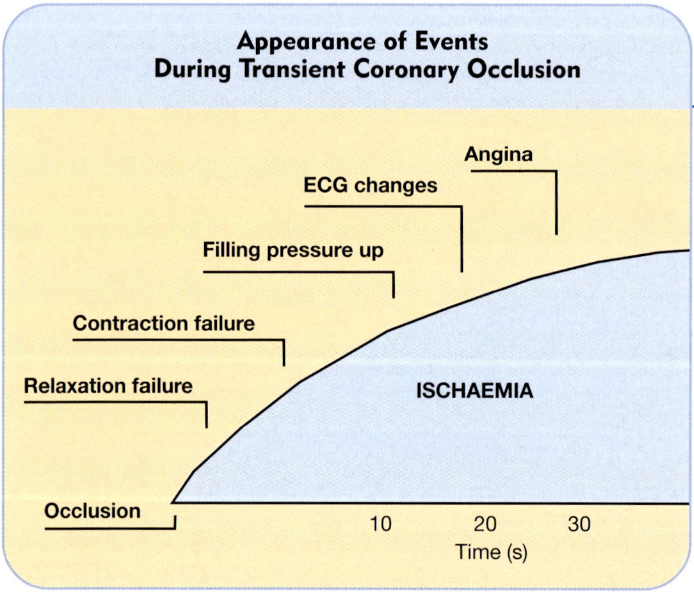

Fig. 8.3 Appearance of events during transient coronary occlusion. Reproduced with kind permission of Springer-Verlag[7].

Characteristics of Stunning, Hibernation, and Ischaemia

Parameter	Stunning	Hibernation	True ischaemia
Myocardial function	Reduced	Reduced	Reduced
Coronary blood flow	Normal/high	Modestly reduced	Most severely reduced
Myocardial energy metabolism	Normal or excessive	Reduced; in steady state	Reduced; increasingly severe as ischaemia proceeds
Duration	Hours to days	Days to hours to months	Minutes to hours
Outcome	Full recovery	Recovery if blood flow restored	Infarction if severe ischaemia persists
Proposed changes in metabolic regulation of calcium	Cystolic overload of calcium in early reperfusion	Just enough glycolytic ATP to prevent contracture	Insufficient glycolytic ATP to prevent irreversibility

Fig. 8.4 Characteristics of stunning, hibernation and ischaemia. Figure adapted from data published in *N Engl J Med*[8].

contractile activity as a direct result of chronic ischaemia when blood flow is modestly reduced. Myocardial stunning may form part of the clinical syndromes of stable and unstable angina, acute MI and left ventricular dysfunction with and without heart failure.

6. How are regions of myocardial ischaemia detected, and how is it treated?

Regions of severely ischaemic or hibernating myocardium may be identified using a variety of imaging techniques. Better understanding of the mechanisms which lead to reduced contraction of cardiac muscle following periods of restricted blood flow may lead to more appropriate treatments. Agents which optimise cardiac energy use towards glucose metabolism and preservation of 'energy pools' (e.g. ATP, creatine phosphate) during ischaemia, and which act independently of and perhaps additionally to antioxidants, calcium antagonists or inotropes, may play an important role in contractile dysfunction.

References

1. Davies MJ, Woolf N. Atherosclerosis: what is it and why does it occur? *Br Heart J* 1993;**69(Suppl.)**:S3–11.
2. van der Wal A, Becker AE. Atherosclerotic plaque rupture-pathologic basis of plaque stability and instability. *Cardiovasc Res* 1999;**41**:334–44.
3. Zeiher AM. Endothelial vasodilator dysfunction: pathogenetic link to myocardial ischaemia or epiphenomenon? *Lancet* 1996;**348**:S1–12.
4. Poole-Wilson PA. Haemodynamic and metabolic consequences of angina and myocardial infarction. In: Fox KM (ed.). *Ischaemic Heart Disease*. Lancaster: MTP Press Ltd,1987:123–48.
5. Stryer L. *Biochemistry*. 4th edn. © 1995, 1998, 1981, 1975: WH Freeman and Company..
6. Roberts R, Morris D, Pratt CM, *et al*. Pathophysiology, recognition, and treatment of acute myocardial infarction and its consequences. In: Schlant RC, Alexander RW (eds). *Hurst's: The Heart*, 8th edn. New York: McGraw Hill Inc., 1994:1107–84.
7. Sigwart U, Grbic M, Payot M, *et al*. Ischemic events during coronary artery baloon occlusion. In: Rutishauser W, Roskmann H (eds). *Silent Myocardial Ischaemia*. Berlin: Springer-Verlag, 1984: 29–36.
8. Epstein SE, Quyyumi AA, Bonow RO. Myocardial ischemia – silent or symptomatic. *N Engl J Med* 1998;**318**:1038–43.
9. Opie LH. Introduction. In: Opie LH (ed.). *Stunning, Hibernation and Calcium in Myocardial Ischemia and Reperfusion*. Boston: Kluwer Academic Publishers,1992:1–3.

9. Investigation of Chest Pain in Suspected Coronary Artery Disease

Richard A Best

1. What are the causes of chest pain?

Angina pectoris
Pulmonary embolism
Pneumothorax
Oesophagitis
Referred pain from spine
Anxiety/tension
Myocardial infarction
Pericarditis
Tachycardia
Peptic ulcer
Costochondritis
Aortic dissection
Pleurisy
Oesophageal tear
Gallstones
Shingles

2. How do we distinguish between them?

From the history: The patient's history should point us near to the mark, but it needs time and critical listening. It also involves a simultaneous balancing of probabilities based on the risk factors described. For example, a 30-year-old woman, previously well, with no risk factors has virtually no chance of having angina, unless she is severely anaemic or has the signs of aortic stenosis. By contrast, a 65-year-old man with risk factors for atheroma is highly likely to have angina, even if the pain is atypical.

Angina is usually a tightness or a heaviness not a pain, and although predictable onset with exertion and offset with rest is typical it is far more worrying when it is unpredictable and at rest. It may be burning or worse after a meal (particularly with exertion), and described in the back, the arms, the jaw, even the abdomen, but radiation to the back of the neck or to specific fingers with paraesthesiae makes it unlikely, as does lack of response to nitroglycerine. Long-standing tightness on exertion correlates with a fibrotic stenosis which is probably stable, but discomfort of short duration, which comes and goes, in a patient with a high probability of coronary disease should be treated with the utmost suspicion, as it may well result from a ruptured plaque. There is no correlation between the severity of angina and the risk from the underlying disease; there is no such thing as mild angina. It is important to decide, therefore, not only whether the pain is cardiac, but also to decide the prognosis (see below).

Stable angina is most often confused with skeletal pain, oesophageal reflux[1], or anxiety/tension[2]; these may be long standing, but they are not usually predictable. Skeletal pain is often positional, may be affected by inspiration, and tends to be momentary or long lasting, while chest tightness due to anxiety tends not to be predictably exertional. Reflux may well be worse at night and relieved by appropriate drugs. Anxiety is often not admitted by the patient and an indirect course of questioning may be required, e.g. "Of course chest pain can be made worse by stress".

From examination: Acute ischaemia can be mimicked by any of the conditions described in the answer to question 1, and examination will help to distinguish them. The physical signs are too extensive to be listed here, but a few points can be made: there are no specific signs of myocardial ischaemia, but historical risk factors, plus evidence of vascular disease, such as bruits, loss of peripheral pulses, or hypertensive or diabetic retinopathy, make it more likely.

Skeletal pain may be reproduced not only by direct pressure or spinal percussion but, more commonly, by passive cervical or thoracic spinal movements prolonged to the extremes of movement for five seconds or so[3]. Shingles rash is often preceded by hyperaesthesia in a root distribution.

3. Which conditions can cause angina?

Coronary artery disease
Right ventricular hypertrophy/overload
Tachycardia
Aortic stenosis
Anaemia
Left ventricular hypertrophy
Thyrotoxicosis

Coronary artery disease is usually atheroma, but includes spasm, vasculitis, small vessel disease (the possible cause of some cases of syndrome X – angina, positive exercise test and normal epicardial coronary arteries on angiography)[4], and the rare anomalous origin of a coronary artery which usually presents in childhood.

Aortic stenosis may be hard to detect when it causes severe left ventricular damage, as the pulse becomes smaller and the murmur quieter as ventricular power declines.

Left ventricular hypertrophy usually results from hypertension or aortic stenosis (and the blood pressure may no longer be raised as systolic function deteriorates), but rarer causes include hypertrophic cardiomyopathy and amyloid, although these rarely present with angina.

Anaemia is very important not only as a treatable cause, but also because if it is due to upper gastrointestinal blood loss, aspirin is contraindicated until the cause is treated successfully, or at least until the risk fully assessed.

Thyrotoxicosis produces a resting tachycardia, but may be missed if the patient is in atrial fibrillation.

Tachycardia, e.g. paroxysmal supra-ventricular tachycardia, may produce chest pain and ST depression, even in young people, and in the absence of coronary disease; this may be due to the release of adenosine.

4. How should possible cardiac chest pain be investigated?

If the pain could be cardiac in origin, then the question is whether it is due to chronic stable ischaemia or unstable ischaemia (or pericarditis, which may also require admission if it results from infarction or the diagnosis is in doubt). Chronic stable ischaemia (the definition of chronic has to be a matter of judgement) can be investigated initially in general practice; tests to exclude a primary cause and to evaluate lipids, and an ECG and referral for stress testing are required. Note that computers are not always good at interpreting an ECG, and no decision should be made purely on the strength of a computer analysis.

Unstable ischaemia needs immediate referral. While the incidence of cardiac death or non-fatal infarction in stable patients is around 2% p.a.[5], it is around 15% in six months in unstable angina[6]. Worryingly, in both groups the majority of incidents occur early so that waiting lists for angiography make a nonsense of ideal care (assuming that intervention can alter outlook for high-risk patients if they can be adequately identified)[7–9]. **Fig. 9.1** presents a suggested way of investigation.

First consider stable angina. Many patients are not referred, but the stress test gives a clue, if a crude one, to prognosis, and to the presence of disease which may best be treated by surgery (although the evidence for this, e.g. the CASS[10] study, predates the advent of statins and angiotensin-converting enzyme inhibitors). Open access stress testing requires a good level of cardiac knowledge from the GP, but chest pain clinics almost by definition, offer same day service and therefore same day stress tests.

Fig. 9.1 provides three options for unstable angina; this might be appropriate for someone with few risk factors, a history of several months and rather unpredictable but ischaemic-sounding pain which therefore does not qualify as stable angina. In the chest pain clinic, if there is no evidence of ongoing ischaemia from the patient's history, resting ECG and troponin T level, stress testing is appropriate and subsequent management depends in part on the results. Any evidence of recent or ongoing ischaemia requires admission, with confirmation of the diagnosis by ECGs during symptoms and after relief (the electrodes should not be moved). Appropriate treatment should be given, almost always with aspirin (consider clopidogrel) and later with heparin, beta-blockers, calcium-antagonists (usually dihydropyridines with a beta-blocker, verapamil or diltiazem without), buccal or intravenous nitrates or nicorandil. The latter has been shown to be safe and protective in unstable ischaemia[11]. If the patient settles, stress testing is appropriate; if not, or if the exercise test is strongly positive, coronary angiography is indicated. It is worth noting in the Vanquwish trial, which showed that routine intervention in unstable angina was associated with an increased mortality in the intervention group, there were no deaths in the angioplasty group, only among the patients who had bypass surgery[9]. Crossover of patients from conservative to aggressive treatment makes the results hard to interpret; further trials are under way.

5. How does response to treatment help in diagnosis?

Nitroglycerine usually relieves angina (although not so readily the pain of infarction) within two to five minutes, and lack of response casts considerable doubt on the diagnosis, as does lack of response to both beta-blockers and calcium antagonists (although lack of response to one class is not so unusual, as might be expected from the different mechanisms of angina). Response to nitroglycerine is not so helpful as it relieves smooth muscle spasm in other organs, and may help musculoskeletal pain. There may be a powerful placebo effect. Lack of response to treatment and absent changes on ECG during pain or stress testing without a clear diagnosis may well lead to coronary angiography, this is useful if it shows no visible disease, but in a population with a high likelihood of atheroma it may just reinforce the patient's worries and lead sometimes to an intervention that does nothing for the symptoms.

6. What is the role of blood tests in the assessment of chest pain?

Apart from the routine full blood count, check of electrolytes, creatinine, lipid and glucose levels, and sometimes TSH and LFTs, biochemical markers of cardiac damage are most frequently useful in the acute situation, i.e. myoglobin (MB), creatine kinase (CK), troponins (Tn) T and I, and sometimes lactate dehydrogenase (LDH).

MB is released earliest when cardiac muscle is damaged; it is a very sensitive but not specific test, and therefore of most use when negative. CK is slower to be detected, but is quite sensitive and where it becomes significantly raised estimation of the percentage which is MB fraction (i.e. of cardiac origin) makes it quite a specific test. The accuracy has been shown in one trial[12] to be increased by also measuring the relative lymphocyte count, which appears to fall in infarction but not with angina. It is the biochemical mainstay of most UK hospitals, but seems likely to be superseded by Tn.

TnT and TnI have both proved useful. Tn is released early and levels may be raised for a week or so, allowing retrospective diagnosis, and superseding the cardiac isoenzyme of LDH which also takes some days to fall. Furthermore it is highly sensitive, identifying patients with unstable angina at higher risk than usual[13], and correlating with inadequate reperfusion[14] and reduced ejection fraction after infarction[15]. It is highly specific and is unaffected by exercise or exercise testing[16,17], and has been used with a normal ECG as a means of identifying patients at very low risk who do not need admission[18]. Rate of rise of CK and TnT gives a guide to infarct artery patency[19]. A normal test six hours after the pain confirms low risk and research continues to see if four hours is as good a discriminant. There is also, however, evidence that CK-MB mass may be a better predictor of infarction in some patients with non-diagnostic ECGs[20]. In trials of new drugs and interventions it is probable that Tn levels will be included as important risk markers.

The white cell count, C-reactive protein, fibrinogen and homocysteine levels may be of interest in epidemiological studies (and fibrinogen levels might prove to be a guide to using warfarin or aspirin), but in terms of assessing an individual with chest pain they are not useful.

7. What is the long-term prognosis of patients with angina pectoris?

In the Framingham study, men with stable angina followed for 14 years had an equal chance of dying or infarcting and about 3.6% p.a. did so; women did twice as well[21]. Twenty years later, with a four-year follow-up, patients on beta-blockers and aspirin had equivalent rates of 0.4% for death and 1% for infarction[6]. The presence of multiple risk factors, particularly previous infarction, and more particularly with unsuccessful reperfusion, low ejection fraction or ventricular arrhythmias, increases risk dramatically and makes accurate individual prognosis impossible, as does the effect of the statins and the fibrates, angiotensin-converting enzyme inhibitors and beta-blockers and the host of drugs and interventions at present under trial. Neither non-invasive testing nor catheterisation gives an unequivocal guide, and the prognostic role of intervention remains uncertain in many situations.

It is worth mentioning the prognosis of patients with chest pain who have been reassured by a cardiologist that they have no evidence of heart disease. The absence of a definite diagnosis has a negative effect in terms of quality of life. Mayou *et al*. showed that many patients remain out of work, and some have been readmitted with chest pain in spite of reassurance that they do not have cardiac pain[22]. Many were regarded as needing psychological help. Of the 50% plus of patients referred to outpatients who do not have symptoms due to ischaemia perhaps a third have been described as being helped by proton pump inhibitors[2], and a similar number have diagnosable skeletal pain[23]. Exclusion of potentially lethal disease, therefore, is not the end of the story.

8. When should a GP refer chest pain patients to a cardiologist?

If the pain is possibly cardiac and the patient is generally fit enough to undergo intervention (30 day mortality for bypass surgery can be as low as 4–5% in the over 70s), referral is needed, particularly where symptoms are acute,

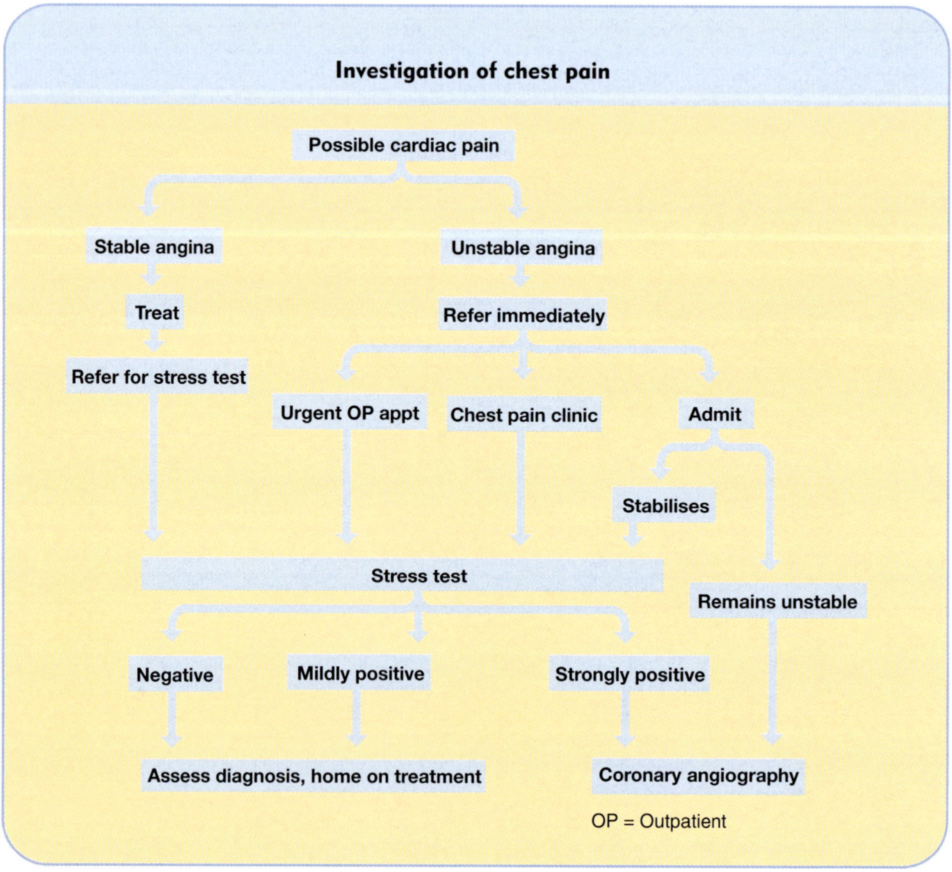

Fig. 9.1 Investigation of chest pain.

unstable or uncontrolled by drugs. In chronic stable angina the GP may find it difficult to exclude aortic stenosis or to decide on lipid lowering. Stress testing may give a clue to mainstem disease, for example, which still merits surgery in most patients since the pre-statin five-year-survival reported in the CASS registry was only 48% in those medically treated; three-vessel disease with a reduced ejection fraction and significant angina was no better, with a survival rate of 52%. The results of surgery have been summarised by Cleland[24]. These patients cannot be identified by their symptoms and therefore specialist cardiological input should be sought.

Guidelines are regularly published and need frequent revision; excellent papers have recently been published on unstable angina[25] and stable angina[26] on behalf of the CESAR group and the British Cardiac Society with the Royal College of Physicians respectively.

References

1. Magarian GJ, Hickham DM. Noncardiac causes of angina-like chest pain. *Prog Cardiovasc Dis* 1986;**29**:65–80.
2. Tew R, Guthrie EA, Creed FH, *et al*. A long-term follow-up study of patients with ischaemic heart disease versus patients with nonspecific chest pain. *J Psychosomatic Res* 1995;**39**:971–5.
3. Yates A. Spondylosis and disc lesions. In: Currey HLF (ed.). *Clinical Rheumatology*. 3rd edn. London: Pittman Medical, 1980:109.
4. Chauhan A, Mullins PA, Gill R, *et al*. Coronary flow reserve and oesophageal in syndrome X. *Postgrad Med J* 1996;**72**:99–104.
5. Juul Moller S, Edvardsson N, Jahnmatz B, *et al*. Double-blind trial of aspirin in primary prevention of myocardial infarction in patients with stable chronic angina pectoris. The Swedish Angina Pectoris Aspirin Trial (SAPAT) Group. *Lancet* 1992;**340**:1421–5.
6. Duncan B. Prognosis of new and worsening angina pectoris. *BMJ* 1976;**1**:981–5.
7. Boden WE, O'Rourke RA, Crawford MH, *et al*. Outcomes in patients with acute non-Q-wave myocardial infarction randomly assigned to an invasive as compared with a conservative management strategy. Veterans Affairs Non-Q-Wave Infarction Strategies in Hospital (VANQWISH) Trial Investigators. *N Engl J Med* 1998;**338**:1785–92.
8. TIMI IIIB Investigators. Effects of tissue plasminogen activator and a comparison of early and invasive and conservative strategies in unstable angina and non-Q-wave myocardial infarction: results of the TIMI IIIB trial. Thrombolysis in myocardial ischaemia. *Circulation* 1994;**89**:1545–56.
9. Lange RA, Hillis LD. Use and overuse of angiography and revascularizarion for acute syndromes. *N Engl J Med* 1998;**338**:1838–9.
10. Yusuf S, Zucker D, Peduzzi P, *et al*. Effect of coronary artery bypass graft surgery on survival: overview of 10-year results from randomised trials by the Coronary Artery Bypass Graft Surgery Trialists Collaboration. *Lancet* 1994;**334**:563–70.
11. Dana A, Yellon DM. Novel cardioprotective agents in acute coronary syndromes: a role for nicorandil? *Br J Cardiol* 1998;**5**:186–7.
12. Thomson SP, Gibbons RJ, Smars PA, *et al*. Incremental value of the leukocyte differential and the rapid creatine kinase-MB isoenzyme for the early diagnosis of myocardial infarction. *Ann Intern Med* 1995;**122**:335–41.
13. Galvani M, Ottani F, Ferrini D, *et al*. Prognostic influence of elevated values of cardiac troponin I in patients with unstable angina. *Circulation* 1997;**95**:2053–9.
14. Sayre MR, Kaufman KH, Chen IW, *et al*. Measurement of cardiac troponin T is an effective method for predicting complications among emergency department patients with chest pain. *Ann Emergency Med* 1998;**31(5)**:539–49.
15. Rao AC, Collinson PO, Canepa-Anson R, *et al*. Troponin T measurement after myocardial infarction can identify left ventricular ejection of less than 40%. *Heart* 1998; **80**:223–5.
16. Collinson PO, Chandler HA, Stubbs PJ, *et al*. Measurement of serum troponin T, creatine kinase MB isoenzyme, and total creatine kinase following arduous physical training. *Ann Clin Biochem* 1995;**32**:450–3.
17. Best RA. Troponin T and exercise testing. *Br J Cardiol;* in press.
18. Hamm CW, Goldmann BU, Heeschen C, *et al*. Emergency room triage of patients with acute chest pain by means of rapid testing for troponin T or troponin I. *N Engl J Med* 1997;**337**:1648–53.
19. Norris RM, Johnson RN, White HD, *et al*. Non-invasive diagnosis of infarct artery patency after acute myocardial infarction by use of serial plasma troponin T concentrations: importance of measurement of peak levels. *Heart* 1996;**75**:481–5.
20. Katz IA, Irwig L, Vinen VD, *et al*. Biochemical markers of acute myocardial infarction: strategies for improving their clinical usefulness. *Ann Clin Biochem* 1998;**35**:393–9.
21. Kannel WB, Sorlie PD. Remission of clinical angina pectoris: the Framingham study. *Am J Cardiol* 1978;**42**:119–23.
22. Mayou R. Invited review: atypical chest pain. *J Psychosomatic Res* 1989;**33**:393–406.
23. Best RA. Non-cardiac chest pain: a new physical sign. *Heart* 1999;**81**:450.
24. Cleland JG. Effect of coronary artery bypass graft surgery on survival. *Lancet* 1994;**344**;1222–4.
25. Patel D. Current diagnostic and therapeutic strategies in unstable angina. *Br J Cardiol* 1999;**6**:80–91
26. De Bono DP, Hopkins A. The investigation and management of stable angina. *J R Coll Physicians Lond* 93;**27**:267–73.

10. The Diagnosis, Treatment and Care of Patients with Myocardial Infarction

Carl Brookes

1. Is there much scope for improvement in the management of myocardial infarction?

Despite the recent reductions in in-hospital mortality following thrombolysis and PTCA, early mortality from myocardial infarction (MI) is still in the region of 30–40%, with 50% of these deaths occurring within the first two hours. These early deaths are mainly due to arrhythmias, predominantly ventricular fibrillation.

There are, therefore, several areas in which improvements in the initial management can be made: reducing the delays in diagnosis, improving early resuscitation and minimising transportation times. These measures require a combination of improved public and patient awareness of the signs and symptoms of acute MI (AMI), training of the general public in basic life-support techniques, and local community arrangements to facilitate urgent transfers.

2. How is a diagnosis of MI made out of hospital?

Taking a good history is vital. The most common symptom is chest pain, usually severe, which lasts longer than 15 minutes and is unresponsive to sub-lingual nitrates. The discomfort is described as constricting or crushing, and is often expressed using a clenched fist held over the sternum. Important other clues include a sense of impending doom and radiation of the pain down the left arm and into the jaw. Some patients, however, have little in the way of pain or discomfort, and in the elderly, in particular, severe chest pain is much less common and AMI may be manifested solely by symptoms of left ventricular failure, profound lethargy or syncope.

The majority of patients with AMI will have evidence of sympathetic activation, with pallor, sweating and tachycardia. Nausea and vomiting occur in over 50%. There are, however, no specific signs of AMI, and both the pulse and blood pressure may be low, normal or high.

If the diagnosis is suspected, an ECG should be obtained as soon as possible. If this requires transfer to hospital then the emergency services should be called immediately. In some countries, general practitioners play a major role in the early care of myocardial infarction, and can initiate reperfusion therapy on the basis of ECG findings in the out-of-hospital setting. In five randomised studies examining this issue, there was a consistent but non-significant trend towards improved outcome in those receiving early out-of-hospital thrombolysis.

3. What proportion of AMIs are silent?

Population based studies suggest that between 20 and 60% of non-fatal AMIs go unrecognised by the patient. Approximately half of these are truly silent and cannot be recalled, even with leading questions. Silent MIs predispose to silent on-going ischaemia. The prognoses for symptomatic and asymptomatic groups appear to be similar.

4. How else is the diagnosis of AMI made?

The advantage of rapid transfer to hospital is that other methods can be used to diagnose AMI. Approximately 40–50% of patients have non-diagnostic ECGs at the time of presentation. Some of these will go on to develop classic ST elevation, but others will not. The development of assays for markers of myocardial injury has helped enormously to establish the diagnosis in these patients. Rapid assays are now available for both the CK-MB isoenzyme of creatine kinase and the cardiac troponins (troponin-T and troponin-I), which allow the detection of myocardial damage within 3–6 hours of onset of chest pain. Serum elevations of the troponins in particular have prognostic implications, and may also have a role in identifying those who fail to reperfuse following treatment[1].

Access to echocardiography is improving, and it is likely that this technique, by identifying regional wall motion abnormalities, will become a useful adjunct in the diagnosis of AMI.

5. Which patients should receive thrombolysis?

More than 100,000 patients have been randomised in thrombolytic trials. For patients presenting within 12 hours of the onset of symptoms the evidence for the benefits of thrombolysis is overwhelming. In all these trials, those patients with a typical history of chest pain and ST elevation of >0.1 mV in two contiguous ECG leads or left bundle branch block, benefit as a group from thrombolysis.

For those treated within 6 hours of symptom onset, approximately 30 deaths per 1000 treated are averted, and for those treated between 7 and 12 hours after symptoms, approximately 20 deaths per 1000 are prevented. Beyond 12 hours there is no convincing evidence of benefit for the group as a whole, although many clinicians would still consider treatment in those with ongoing symptoms and persistent ST elevation[2].

The largest absolute benefit is seen in those at highest risk, i.e. those over 65 years, those presenting with a systolic pressure of <100 mmHg, those with anterior infarction or those with evidence of extensive ischaemia.

Thrombolytic therapy should not be given to patients with ST depression or those with minor ST–T changes.

6. What are the hazards of thrombolysis?

The main concern relates to cerebral haemorrhage, which occurs with an overall incidence of 0.75%. Risks are increased in those >65 years of age, those weighing <70kg, those with systolic hypertension at presentation, and in those who receive front-loaded (accelerated) tissue plasminogen activator (tPA) as opposed to streptokinase (SK). These bleeds lead to an excess risk of approximately four strokes per 1000 patients treated – two fatal and two non-fatal.

Other major non-cerebral bleeds, requiring transfusion or that are life-threatening, occur in about 7 per 1000 treated.

Hypotension can be expected in up to 10% of patients treated with SK, but severe allergic reactions are very uncommon, occurring in approximately 1% of cases.

7. Is there any difference between thrombolytic agents?

When compared with SK, accelerated tPA results in improved rates of reperfusion, particularly when given early after the onset of symptoms, but this is at the expense of a greater risk of intracranial haemorrhage. In the GUSTO I trial there was a small but significant mortality benefit with tPA over SK – 7.2 versus 7.9%. This benefit becomes greater in those patients with a greater baseline risk of mortality.

It must be remembered, however, that many more lives would be saved if it could be ensured that every eligible patient with an AMI received some form of thrombolysis; the exact thrombolytic regime is of relatively little importance.

8. Is there a role for percutaneous transluminal coronary angioplasty (PTCA)?

The advantage of PTCA is that it enables rapid reperfusion of the infarct vessel without the bleeding risks of thrombolysis. The disadvantage is that it is not readily available without introducing significant time delays into the treatment protocol.

In those trials that have compared primary PTCA with thrombolysis at experienced centres, there is a significant prognostic benefit with PTCA – mortality is reduced to <5%. These results are only achievable, however, if a fully staffed 24-hour interventional service can be provided and this is not a realistic option for the UK at the present time.

Under current guidelines, PTCA should be considered in those patients who have contraindications to thrombolysis, those who fail to reperfuse following thrombolysis (rescue PTCA) and, probably, in those who present with or develop cardiogenic shock.

9. Which prophylactic drugs should be used in the acute phase?

There are very few contraindications to aspirin and all patients with an acute coronary syndrome should be carefully considered for aspirin therapy. It has an additive effect in those receiving thrombolysis, resulting in a 42% reduction in mortality.

In those with a true contraindication to aspirin other anti-platelet therapies should be considered, although none has been well tested. Clopidogrel, an ADP-receptor antagonist, is well tolerated and has been shown to be as effective as aspirin in the secondary prevention of cardiovascular events. There is no role at present for the use of prophylactic anti-arrhythmic drugs.

Most of the data relating to beta-blocker therapy in AMI predate the use of thrombolysis. Little data exist on definite benefits since. A pragmatic case, however, can be made for the use of beta-blockers in those patients with a persistent tachycardia without hypotension or heart failure, or those with recurrent ischaemic pain. There is increasing evidence that beta-blockers have a role in the management of patients with chronic heart failure, but these agents should not be introduced in the acute stages.

The routine use of nitrates has not been shown to be of convincing value.

Trials of ACE inhibitor therapy have shown that treatment in the early phase following AMI results in 4.6 fewer deaths per 1000 treated. These drugs are usually started on day 2–4 as a low dose oral preparation. It is likely that these benefits are of particular value in those patients with LV dysfunction or heart failure.

Routine use of magnesium is probably not warranted, but it may be of value in certain subgroups.

10. How should those patients without ST elevation be managed?

In the absence of contraindications, all such patients should be treated as an unstable coronary syndrome with aspirin, heparin and beta-blockers. Continuing pain should be treated with nitrates and opiates. It the pain persists despite treatment or recurs, then referral for PTCA or surgery should be considered to minimise the risks of further myocardial damage.

The ISIS-2, GISSI and TIMI IIIB trials have all failed to show a benefit with thrombolysis in this group of patients[3].

11. What is the prognosis of patients with non-Q wave MIs?

The in-hospital mortality of patients with a non-Q MI is lower (at about 2–3%) than for those with a Q-wave MI, but rates converge over time and are similar at approximately three years. Many people consider that a non-Q MI is an infarct-in-waiting, and this is borne out by the finding that further adverse cardiovascular events occur in 8–10% within six weeks. Risk stratification therefore becomes paramount.

12. How should post-MI patients be managed in hospital?

Most patients should remain in bed for 12–24 hours, but can normally start walking the next day. Those with heart failure or significant arrhythmias should be kept in bed longer. An echocardiogram should be performed to document LV function and to exclude a large intraventricular thrombus requiring anticoagulation.

Recurrent angina at rest or at low levels of activity requires further investigation with coronary angiography. Late ventricular arrhythmias also require further evaluation as revascularisation and/or defibrillator implantation may be necessary.

Prior to discharge, some assessment of future risk should be made (**Figs 10.1** & **10.2**). This is usually based on a mixture of clinical findings, echocardiography and the results of a sub-maximal exercise test. It helps to plan further investigations, improves patient confidence and enables a rehabilitation programme to be constructed.

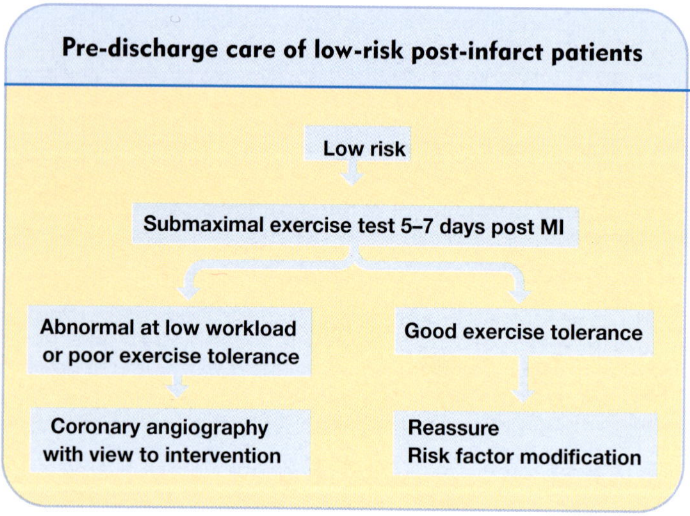

Fig. 10.1 Pre-discharge care of low-risk post-infarct patients.

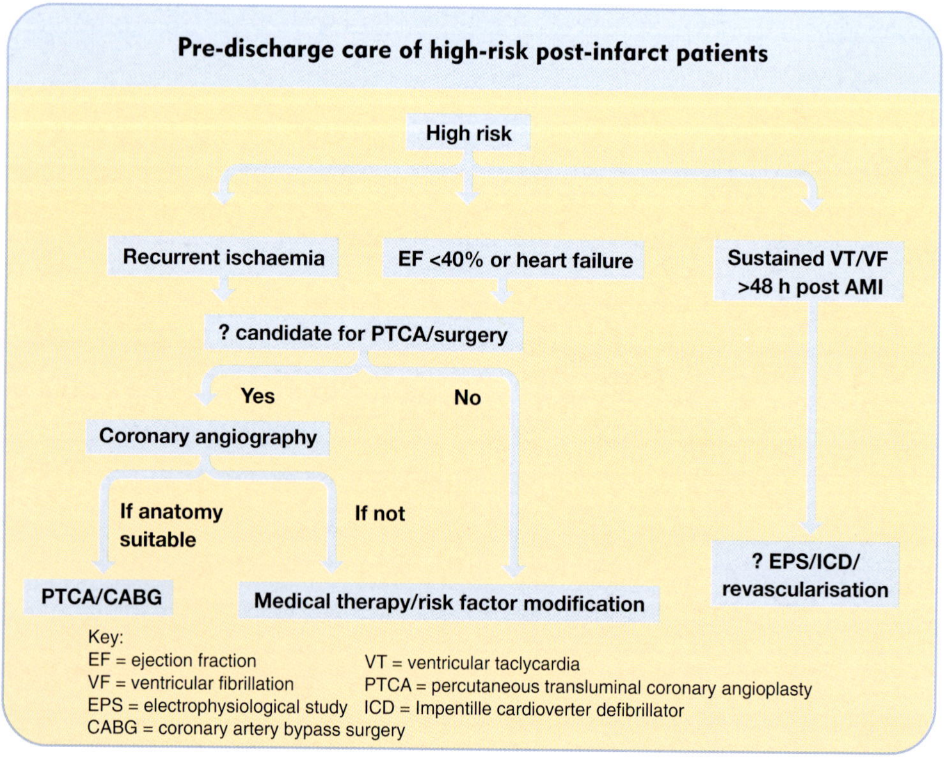

Fig. 10.2 Pre-discharge care of high-risk post-infarct patients.

13. Which factors determine long-term survival?

Left ventricular function, residual ischaemic myocardium and the potential for developing ventricular arrhythmias. LV function should be assessed using echocardiography as the ejection fraction has significant prognostic implications. Exercise testing adds important information, as those with a better exercise tolerance have a better long-term outcome for the same ejection fraction.

Detection of ischaemia is best performed using exercise testing. Those who are unable to carry out a stress test or who have failed to complete stage II of the Bruce protocol, because of symptoms, ECG changes or blood pressure fall, are at high risk[4].

Routine non-invasive screening for potential arrhythmias is of limited predictive value and, at the time of writing, is probably not justified. In the absence of symptoms or the development of arrhythmias during exercise testing, further investigations are not warranted.

14. Which measures are effective in secondary prevention?

There is compelling evidence from observational studies that cessation of smoking reduces the risk of reinfarction by up to 50%. If patients cease smoking their risk becomes similar to that in those who have never smoked within three years. A healthy diet and weight reduction in obese patients is important.

Anti-platelet agents, especially aspirin, reduce death or reinfarction by 25% and should be given to all those without contraindications. Further data on the use of anticoagulants in combination with aspirin following AMI are awaited. At present, the indications for prescribing these agents are:

1. Mural thrombus seen on echocardiography.
2. A large regional wall motion abnormality.
3. Atrial fibrillation.
4. A left ventricular aneurysm.

Beta-blockers reduce the incidence of death or reinfarction by 20–25%. Opinion is divided on whether these drugs should be given to everyone or only those at moderate/high risk.

Trials of verapamil and diltiazem have shown a reduction in events when given post-MI but these drugs should not be used in patients with impaired LV function. They should be considered in those with contraindications to beta-blocker therapy.

There is a strong case for administering ACE inhibitors in patients who have developed heart failure, even if this is only transient, or those with an ejection fraction of less than 40%. In low-risk patients with a normal ejection fraction these agents can be discontinued at 4–6 weeks.

All patients recovering from AMI should be considered for modification of their lipid profile. This will include a diet low in saturated fat, weight reduction and exercise, but often also requires lipid lowering therapy. The 4S study recruited patients at least six months following infarction with a total cholesterol of 5.5–8.0 mmol/l and demonstrated a mortality benefit with simvastatin over placebo. This benefit translated to 33 lives saved per 1000 patients treated. A number of trials have since confirmed the place of the HMG-CoA reductase inhibitors in secondary prevention, and patients who fulfil these criteria should receive these drugs. It is still not clear, however, how soon after infarction therapy should be started.

References

1. Hamm CW. New serum markers for acute myocardial infarction. *N Engl J Med* 1994;**331**:607–9.
2. Task Force on the Management of AMI of the ESC. Acute myocardial infarction: pre-hospital and in-hospital management. *Eur Heart J* 1996;**17**:43–63.
3. TIMI-IIIB Investigators. Effects of tPA and a comparison of early invasive and conservative strategies in unstable angina and non-Q-wave infarction. *Circulation* 1994;**89**:1545–56.
4. Villella A, Maggioni AP, Villella M, *et al*. Prognostic significance of maximal exercise testing after myocardial infarction treated with thrombolytic agents: the GISSI-2 data base. *Lancet* 1995;**346**:523–9.

11. Coronary Risk Factors and Possibilities for Modification

Henry Purcell
Sam Kaddoura

1. How do European heart disease rates compare with those of other developed countries and are things improving or getting worse?

Heart and circulatory disease remains the number one killer in most developed countries[1]. Coronary heart disease (CHD) is the leading cause of death in men over 45 years and women over 65 years throughout Europe.

CHD is manifest clinically as angina pectoris, invariably resulting from atherosclerosis and the development of myocardial ischaemia. An estimated 6.2 million Americans and over 1.5 million Britons have angina. It is primarily a disease of middle age, occurring especially in people in their fifties, but risk rises progressively with increasing age. In the childbearing years women have only about one-quarter the risk of developing CHD compared to men of comparable age, but after 75 years mortality rates are approximately equal between the sexes. While there is no sharp upturn in CHD rates after the menopause[2], women may have relative protection premenopausally from CHD because of the beneficial influence of oestrogens on serum lipids and blood pressure. But ultimately, almost twice as many women die from heart and circulatory disease as they do from cancer.

Prognosis in angina is not benign, as one in 10 cases will experience a non-fatal MI or coronary death within one year of presentation[3]. To put this into a local perspective, a general practitioner with a list of 2000 patients will have five patients die from CHD annually.

In the UK disease rates are still among the highest in the world, where almost half of all individuals die from cardiovascular causes, with 1 in 4 men and 1 in 5 women having a fatal myocardial infarction[4]. Although more than 1 in 5 males and females in the US have some form of cardiovascular disease, and as many as 1.5 million Americans will have a new or recurrent MI every year, there has been a dramatic decline in the CHD death rate of 42% between 1963 (the peak year) and 1985. However, according to new figures which take into account the ageing population, an increase in CHD deaths has recently been reported as the percentage of individuals over 65 has risen.

There is convincing evidence that medical care, ranging from interventions to reduce risk factors, to medical and surgical management of acute and chronic CHD, to resuscitation for cardiac arrest, has accounted for many of the lives saved since CHD mortality peaked. Other developed countries have experienced a decline in CHD. Between the years 1981 and 1991 the fall in death rates in the US among men aged 35 to 74 years was 31%, with a 41% fall in Australia and 35% in Japan (**Fig. 11.1**). In the UK, however, the trend was less marked at 24%. There are also regional differences among the British population, where the premature CHD death rate for men living in the north of England is 37% higher than in the south-east and 81% higher for women living in the north.

Regional differences are also apparent throughout Europe, where rates are lowest in the Mediterranean region and highest in Eastern and Central Europe. Countries such as Hungary and Romania are now highest in the international CHD league table. There is growing concern among health workers about the current epidemic of heart disease in the former Eastern bloc (and the impending epidemic in the Third World), which has occurred over a period of social and economic turmoil and is associated with increased rates of smoking particularly. This has been addressed in the recommendations of the Second Joint Task Force of European and other Societies on Coronary Prevention[5].

2. Is cardiovascular risk factor intervention still the best way forward to prevent heart disease, and what 'new' risk factors have been identified?

The concept of 'risk factors' came from the Framingham Study. A risk factor is defined as a factor associated with either a disease or a condition which is suspected as being causative. As described above, age and gender are strong determinants of CHD, but it has long been recognised that it clusters in families, which may be because these individuals share not only the same genes but eat from a common kitchen and have similar lifestyles. Research towards a better understanding of the genetic susceptibility to atherosclerosis is rapidly advancing, but there are huge gaps in our knowledge, and about half of all patients with CHD do not have any of the established risk factors, i.e. hypertension, hypercholesterolaemia, cigarette smoking, diabetes, marked obesity and physical inactivity[6].

There are a number of new 'candidate' risk factors, including infectious agents such as *Chlamydia pneumoniae* and specific agents influencing endothelial function and blood coagulation, including homocysteine and fibrinogen. However, there are a number of clearly established risk factors that can help identify 'at risk' individuals. CHD is multifactorial, as is its treatment and prevention, and it is likely that much can be done by impacting on the 'Big Three' factors: dyslipidaemia, smoking and hypertension.

Dyslipidaemia

There is a strong correlation between high serum cholesterol concentrations, development of atherosclerosis and the clinical occurrence of CHD. The Multiple Risk Factor Intervention Trial (MRFIT) was one of the early observational

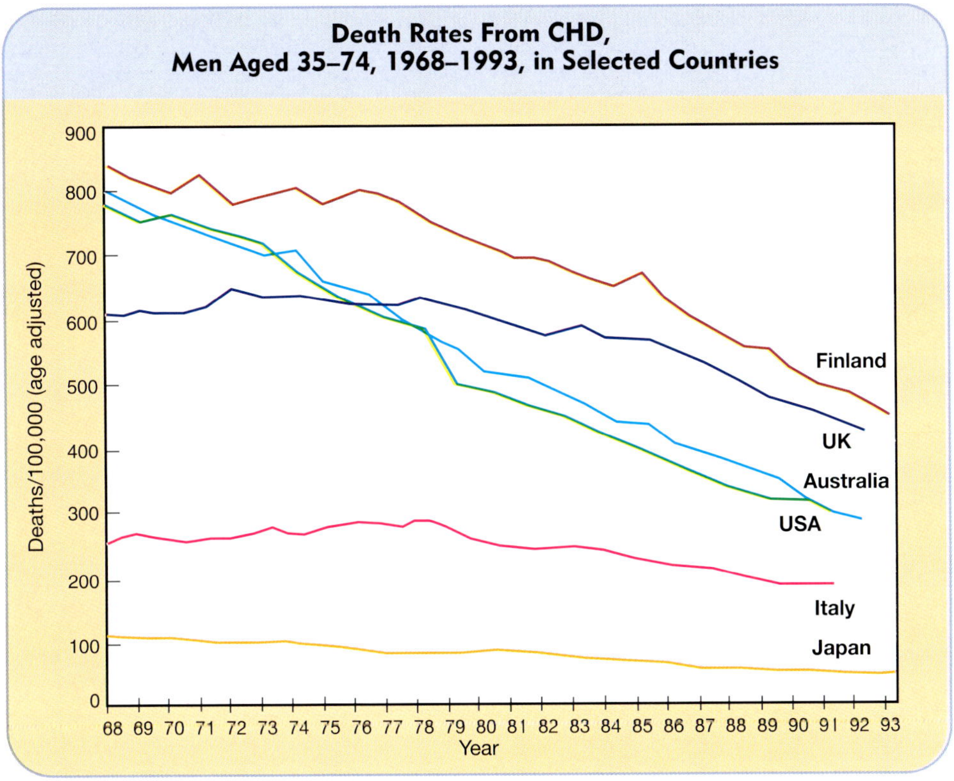

Fig. 11.1 Death rates from coronary heart disease in men aged 35–74 years (1968–1993) in selected countries Reproduced with kind permission from the British Heart Foundation[4].

population studies to show the risk of CHD is strong and continuous over the whole range of serum cholesterol concentration, with risk increasing substantially when the cholesterol exceeds 6.5 mmol/l[7]. Similarly, in populations with higher mean cholesterol levels (such as in Northern Europe and North America) CHD is responsible for about half of all deaths, in contrast to countries like Japan and some Mediterranean regions, where lower cholesterols are associated with lower CHD mortality. A number of intervention trials conducted in the 1980s with lipid-lowering drugs such as bile acid sequestrants, e.g. cholestyramine, fibrates, gemfibrozil, showed that reducing cholesterol had a beneficial effect on non-fatal and fatal CHD events[8]. The gain appeared to be that for every 1% reduction in cholesterol there was a 2% reduction in CHD risk. To obtain a reduction in total mortality, however, plasma cholesterol needs to be reduced by more than a modest 5–10%. The HMG-CoA reductases (statins) can lower cholesterol by 20–25%, and trials have now been conducted which confirm the clinical benefits in patients with CHD. The most intensively investigated agents are simvastatin and pravastatin.

The 'landmark' statin trial was the Scandinavian Simvastatin Survival Study (4S) [9]. In the 4S, some 4444 patients with angina or previous MI (79%) who had a serum cholesterol between 5.0 and 8.0 mmol/l on a lipid-lowering diet were randomised to double-blind treatment with simvastatin or placebo. Over the 5.4 year median follow-up period there was a 30% decrease in total mortality in the simvastatin treated group, which was attributable to a 42% decrease in CHD deaths. CHD incidence fell by 33% and the need for revascularisation was reduced by 37%. The risk of new or worsening intermittent claudication, bruits and angina pectoris was also reduced by simvastatin. These effects are consistent with the statin trials showing reductions also in cerebrovascular events, suggesting that retardation of progression of atherosclerosis is not limited to the coronary vasculature. Simvastatin improved survival in patients aged 60 or more and reduced major coronary events in women (about 19% of the study population) by about the same extent as it did in men. All of these benefits have been shown to be maintained for up to eight years.

There have been several further trials of statins since 4S. The West of Scotland Coronary Prevention Study (WOSCOPS)[10] was a primary prevention trial conducted in males with hypercholesterolaemia (mean cholesterol 7.0 mmol/l) randomised to treatment with pravastatin or placebo for an average follow-up period of 4.9 years. The Air Force/Texas coronary atherosclerosis prevention study (AF/TexCAPS) also looked at primary prevention, in 5608 middle-aged men and 997 women (mean total cholesterol 5.7 mmol/l), randomised to lovastatin or placebo and followed up over seven years. It had the power to cause a reduction in new events only[11]. The cholesterol and recurrent events trial (CARE)[12] enrolled men and women (14% women) with mean serum cholesterol levels <6.2 mmol/l, 3–20 months post-myocardial infarction. They were randomised to pravastatin or placebo and followed for an average of five years. And, the Long-Term Intervention with Pravastatin in Ischaemic Disease Study (LIPID)[13] randomised men and women (17% women) with a median cholesterol of 5.6 mmol/l who had had a myocardial infarction (MI) or unstable angina 3 to 36 months earlier to treatment with pravastatin or placebo for a mean follow-up period of 6.1 years.

The key findings from these studies are summarised in **Fig. 11.2**[14]. These provide long-term support for the safety and efficacy of lipid-lowering drug therapy in patients who are 'at risk' for CHD and who have failed to respond to dietary therapy. This benefit extends to those individuals, male or female, young or older patients, with a history of MI and angina or with no evidence of prior MI as in WOSCOPS (but 5% had evidence of angina) where enrolment was restricted to males. Statins have been shown to reduce myocardial ischaemia, and may cause stabilisation of atherosclerotic plaques that are prone to rupture. Several mechanisms of plaque stabilisation are under investigation. These include:

Antithrombotic/antiplatelet mechanisms
Anti-inflammatory/antioxidant mechanisms
Restoration of endothelial function.

Smoking

In the USA, nearly 1 in 5 deaths from cardiovascular diseases are attributable to smoking. Non-fatal MI rates are five times as great among cigarette smokers as among non-smokers at ages 30–49, three times as great at ages 50–59 and twice as great at ages 60–79[15]. It is worrying, therefore, that the incidence of daily use of cigarettes increased by 50% among 12–17 year old Americans between 1988 and 1996. Similarly in the UK, rates are increasing among the young but 1997 figures show that overall, 28% of women and 29% of men are smokers. Smoking remains the largest single preventable cause of death and disability, accounting for more that 120,000 deaths annually. Many studies have shown that smoking cessation treatment works[16].

Hypertension

Hypertension is also one of the most prevalent and powerful contributors to CHD deaths, increasing risk on average two- to three-fold[17]. Hypertension clusters with dyslipidaemia, insulin resistance, glucose intolerance and obesity, occurring in isolation in less than 20% of cases. The heart is a target organ in the presence of sustained high arterial blood pressure, and development of left ventricular hypertrophy (LVH), an ominous harbinger of cardiovascular disease, increases risk of development of heart failure and sudden death dramatically. Reducing hypertension reduces risk of both stroke and CHD.

Clearly, every effort must be made to control these and other cardiovascular risk factors in order to improve prognosis in patients with angina.

3. How can cardiovascular risk be measured?

Framingham workers have recently calculated that lifetime risk of developing CHD at age 40 years is 1 in 2 for men and 1 in 3 for women[18]. Even at age 70 years it is 1 in 3 for men and 1 in 4 for women. These figures validate the need to educate, screen, and treat for prevention of CHD in younger and older patients.

A number of calculators, computer programs and other devices utilising Framingham data are available to help measure the cardiovascular risk in an individual. One of the simplest, however, is the Modified New Zealand Risk

'Statin' Trials

	Trial	Number	% Reduction in TC	% Risk reduction (primary end-point)
Secondary prevention	4S	4444	–25	–30 (total mortality) $P = 0.0003$
	CARE	4159	–20	–24 (CHD death/non-fatal MI) $P = 0.003$
	LIPID	9014	–18	–24 (CHD death) $P < 0.001$
Primary prevention	WOSCOPS	6595	–20	–31 (CHD death/non-fatal MI) $P < 0.001$

Fig. 11.2 Evidence from trials in patients (**a**) with established heart disease (secondary prevention), and (**b**) without overt coronary heart disease (primary prevention).

Table (**Fig. 11.3**)[19] which help estimate the absolute risk of developing a cardiovascular event (MI, new angina, stroke, or transient ischaemic event), for a wide range of ages and include total cholesterol:high density lipoprotein cholesterol ratios.

4. Is there any clear evidence that a national policy of cardiovascular risk factor intervention can reduce CHD mortality?

Yes. In the early 1970s Finland had the highest CHD mortality in the world. They then implemented a national strategy to reduce CHD, mainly by reducing the levels of known risk factors in the population. The observed changes in risk factors from 1972 to 1992 predicted a 43% decline in CHD mortality in men and a 49% decline in women. The actual changes were 55% and 68% respectively (**Fig. 11.4**). Most of this decline can be explained by changes in the three main coronary risk factors, dyslipidaemia, smoking and hypertension[20]. Up to half of the recent large falls in CHD mortality rates in New Zealand are attributed to medical therapies, while half are also attributed to reductions in major risk factors.[21]

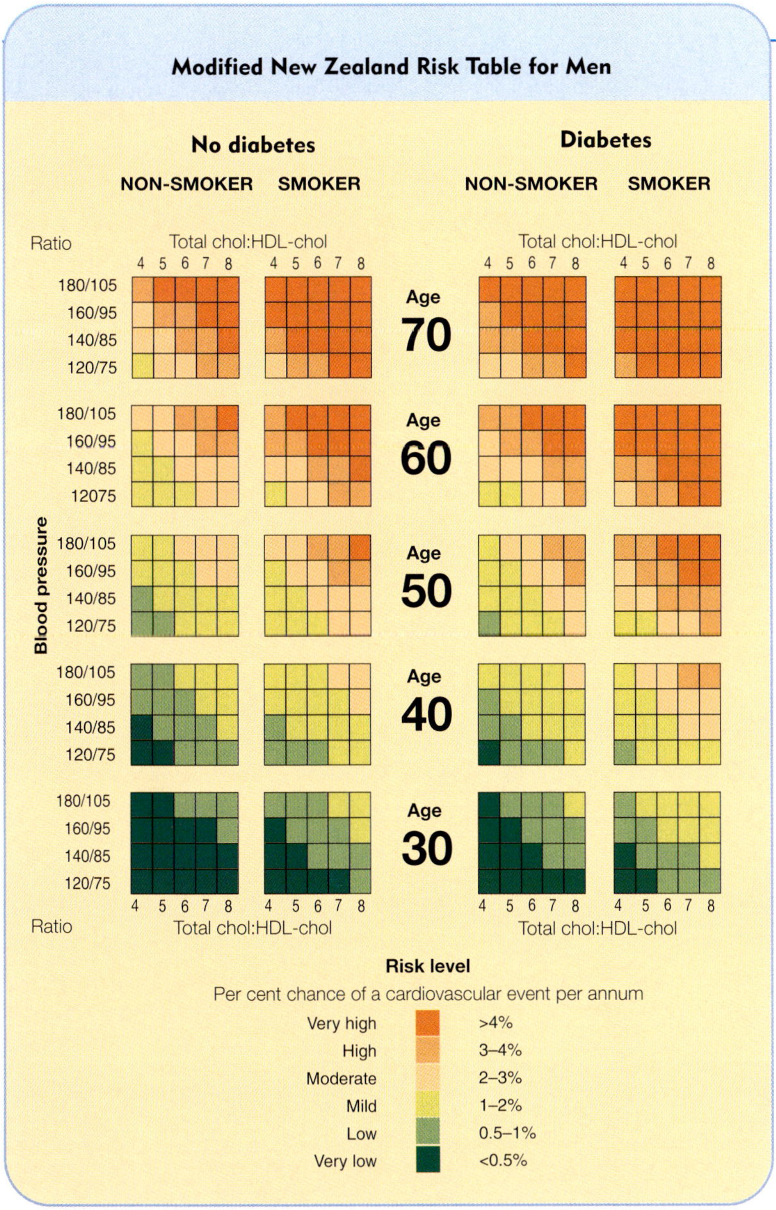

Fig. 11.3 Coronary Risk Chart. Reproduced with kind permission of the BMJ Publishing Group[19].

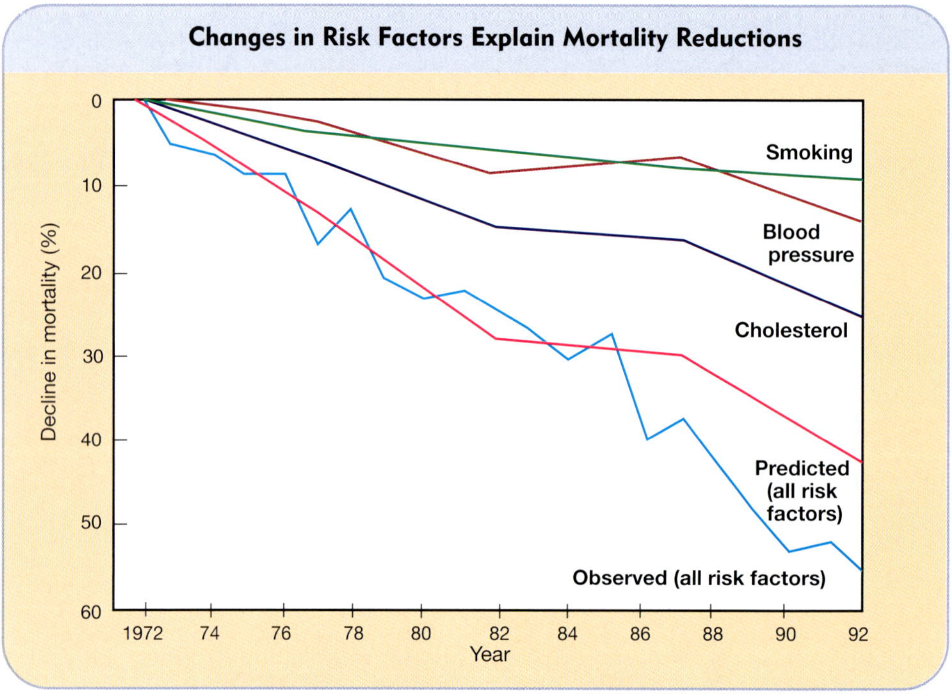

Fig. 11.4 Observed and predicted decline in coronary heart disease mortality in men in Finland (1972–92). Reproduced with kind permission of the BMJ Publishing Group[20].

References

1. 1999 Heart and Stroke Statistical Update. Dallas: American Heart Association, 1999 (www.americanheart.org).
2. Khaw K-T. Epidemiology of coronary heart disease in women. In: Julian D, Wenger NK (eds). *Women and Heart Disease*. London: Martin Dunitz, 1997:7–20.
3. Gandhi M, Lampe FC, Wood DA. Incidence, clinical characteristics, and short-term prognosis of angina pectoris. *Br Heart J* 1995;**73**:193–8.
4. British Heart Foundation. Coronary heart disease statistics. British Heart Foundation Statistics Database. London: BHF, 2000.
5. Prevention of coronary heart disease in clinical practice. Recommendations of the Second Joint Task Force of European and other Societies on Coronary Prevention. *Eur Heart J* 1998;**19**:1434–503.
6. Braunwald E. Shattuck lecture – cardiovascular medicine at the turn of the millennium: Triumphs, concerns, and opportunities. *N Engl J Med* 1997;**337**:1360–9.
7. Grundy SM. Cholesterol and coronary heart disease. A new era. *J Am Med Assoc* 1986;**256**:2849–58.
8. Holme I. Relation of coronary heart disease incidence and total mortality to plasma cholesterol reduction in randomised trials:use of meta-analysis. *Br Heart J* 1993;**69(Suppl.)**:S42–S47.
9. Scandinavian Simvastatin Survival Study Group. Randomised trial of cholesterol lowering in 444 patients with coronary heart disease; the Scandinavian Simvastatin Survival Study (4S). *Lancet* 1994;**344**:1383–9.
10. Shepherd J, Cobbe SM, Ford I, *et al*. Prevention of coronary heart disease with pravastatin in men with hypercholesterolemia. *N Engl J Med* 1995;**333**:1301–7.
11. Downs JR, Clearfield M, Whitney E, *et al*. Air Force/Texas coronary atherosclerosis prevention study (AFCAPS/TexCAPS). *J Am Med Assoc* 1998;**279**:1615–22.
12. Sacks FM, Pfeffer MA, Moye LA, *et al*. The effect of pravastatin on coronary events after myocardial infarction in patients with average cholesterol values. *N Engl J Med* 1996;**335**:1001–9.
13. The Long-Term Intervention with Pravastatin in Ischaemic Disease (LIPID) Study Group. Prevention of cardiovascular events and death with pravastatin in patients with coronary heart disease and a broad range of initial cholesterol levels. *N Engl J Med* 1998;**339**:1349–57.
14. Wierzbicki A. When should statins be prescribed? *Update* 1998;**7 October**:476–90.
15. Parish S, Collins R, Peto R, *et al*. Cigarette smoking, tar yields, and non-fatal myocardial infarction: 14 000 cases and 32 000 controls in the United Kingdom. *Br Med J* 1995;**311**:471–7.
16. Hughes JR, Goldstein MG, Hurt RD, Shiffman S. Recent advances in the pharmacotherapy of smoking. *J Am Med Assoc* 1999;**281**:72–6.
17. Kannel WB. Blood pressure as a cardiovascular risk factor. Prevention and treatment. *J Am Med Assoc* 1996;**275**:1571–6.
18. Lloyd-Jones DM, Larson MG, Beiser A, Levy D. Lifetime risk of developing coronary heart disease. *Lancet* 1999;**353**:89–92.
19. McLeod AJ, Armitage M. Use of Statins. But New Zealand tables are better. *BMJ* 1998;**317**:474
20. Vartiainen E, Puska P, Pekkanen J, *et al*. Changes in risk factors explain changes in mortality from ischaemic heart disease in Finland. *Br Med J* 1994;**309**:23–7.
21. Capewell S, Beaglehole R, Seddon M, McMurray J. Explanation for the decline in coronary heart disease mortality rates in Auckland, New Zealand, between 1982–1993. *Circulation* 2000;**102**:1511–16.

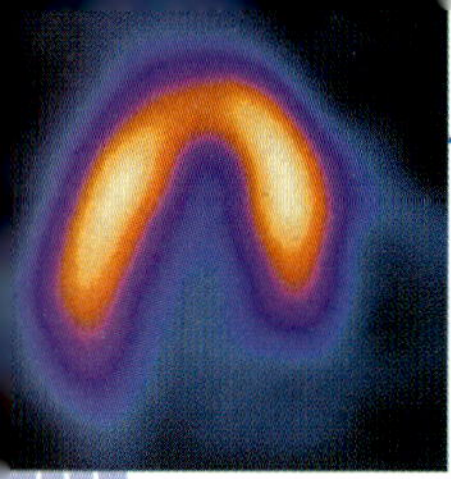

III. Patient Populations

12. Women

Diana R Holdright

1. What are the risks of women developing coronary artery disease?

Breast cancer is the major health concern among women, despite the fact that coronary artery disease is by far the greater killer in the Western world. The frequently quoted breast cancer figure of 1 in 12 is misleading since it represents the risk of *younger* women *developing*, rather than *dying* from, breast cancer. The *lifetime* risk of *dying* from breast cancer is far less – 1 in 24 for a 30 year old and 1 in 30 for a 60 year old. In stark contrast, the lifetime risk of dying from coronary artery disease is 1 in 3.4 for a 30 year old woman and 1 in 3.3 for a 60 year old.

2. What are the major cardiovascular risk factors in women?

Cardiovascular risk factors are generally similar for men and women. For example, total cholesterol, HDL cholesterol, triglycerides and systolic blood pressure are among the most important risk factors for both sexes[1]. However, there are exceptions, and even if relative risks for a given risk factor are similar, the absolute risks will be lower in women than in men.

The lipid profile changes considerably with age in women, particularly after the menopause, when HDL cholesterol falls and LDL cholesterol, triglycerides and Lp(a) rise. Consequently, a full lipid profile should be obtained in all patients and not simply a measure of total cholesterol. Compared with men, the ratio of total to HDL cholesterol is a far more reliable discriminator of the presence of coronary artery disease in women than total cholesterol alone. There is increasing evidence that raised triglycerides are a risk factor for heart disease, and that this is more so in women.

Hypertension, a major risk factor for stroke, heart failure and ischaemic heart disease, is more common in older women than men. Left ventricular hypertrophy is a greater cardiovascular risk in women. Diabetes mellitus is a far greater risk factor in women, completely removing the gender advantage. Death rates from coronary artery disease are 3–7 times greater in diabetic women than in non-diabetic women, compared with a 2–4 fold difference in men.

Cigarette smoking, which is the leading preventable cause of death in developed countries, is a greater risk factor for myocardial infarction in women than in men. This gender difference is difficult to explain, but women smokers are relatively oestrogen deficient. Currently, more teenage girls than boys smoke. Smoking quadruples the risk of coronary artery disease in women; even light smokers of 1 to 4 cigarettes/day double their risk. The combination of smoking plus another risk factor greatly increases risk, e.g. the relative risk of ischaemic heart disease in a diabetic woman smoker is 22.3 compared with a non-diabetic non-smoker.

3. What is the role of oestrogen in coronary artery disease?

The incidence of coronary artery disease rises after the menopause, partly due to ageing but also due to the loss of protective endogenous oestrogens. Potential cardioprotective mechanisms include a favourable alteration of the lipid profile, vasodilator properties and antioxidant effects. Meta-analyses of older trials suggested a 40–50% reduction in coronary artery disease with hormone replacement therapy (HRT) in postmenopausal women. However, the recently published HERS trial, which is the first prospective, randomised placebo-controlled double blind study of HRT in postmenopausal women suggested no overall cardiovascular benefit from HRT[2]. Moreover, there were significantly more thromboembolic events in women taking HRT compared with placebo.

This trial, at odds with the majority of earlier publications, has created considerable confusion but it can be criticised on several counts – for the HRT preparation chosen (not the most 'cardiovascular friendly' or the preferred type in Europe), for the age of the patients treated (an average of 15 years past the menopause) and for the short duration of the trial (4.1 years), which mechanistically is probably not long enough to see any significant potential benefit from treatment. Indeed, there was a time trend towards benefit in the later years of treatment.

In an attempt to summarise, HRT should be prescribed for postmenopausal symptoms but not for secondary prevention of coronary artery disease as the main indication. Whether or not there is real cardiovascular benefit is uncertain. Trials of primary prevention are in progress. Interest has now turned to the new selective oestrogen receptor modulator drugs, such as raloxifene, which have beneficial effects on bone density and the lipid profile without adverse effects on the uterus or breast, in contrast to unopposed oestrogen therapy[3]. Whether they will have a protective effect on the heart remains to be seen.

4. Do women with ischaemic heart disease present differently to men?

Nearly half of all women present with angina as the initial manifestation of ischaemic heart disease. In contrast, myocardial infarction is the initial presentation in nearly 50% of men. Women are older at first presentation by up to 10 years and they generally have a worse risk factor profile and greater comorbidity. Women have higher total cholesterol levels, and a greater incidence of diabetes and hypertension, but are less likely to have a history of cigarette smoking, although this may change in future years. Comparing the different modes of presentation among women, those presenting with angina tend to be younger than women presenting with myocardial infarction, and they tend to have more favourable risk factor profiles.

Importantly, women presenting with angina not only have more favourable risk factor profiles but they also have a better prognosis compared with women with other initial presentations of heart disease and compared with men[4]. The findings of angiographic studies suggest that a proportion of women with a clinical diagnosis of angina actually have normal coronary arteries, which probably explains the different risk factor profile and better prognosis in this subgroup. Atypical chest pain is more common in women than in men and identification of those women with ischaemic heart disease is more difficult[5].

5. What are the causes of chest pain in women?

Many studies have shown a higher incidence of angiographically normal coronary arteries in women catheterised because of chest pain compared with men. Undoubtedly, in some cases there may still be a cardiac explanation for the pain. Left ventricular hypertrophy secondary to severe hypertension or aortic stenosis may give rise to myocardial ischaemia. Syndrome X and microvascular angina (see below) are also possibilities, although uncommon.

There is a high incidence, in some series as high as 60%, of oesophageal abnormalities in patients with chest pain and angiographically normal coronary arteries. Nutcracker oesophagus, diffuse oesophageal spasm and non-specific motility disorders have all been described. Oesophageal reflux is an important and common differential diagnosis. Acid reflux has even been shown to reduce coronary blood flow, which is a putative mechanism for producing cardiac pain[6]. Musculoskeletal causes of chest pain should also be considered.

6. What are syndrome X and microvascular angina? Do they matter?

Syndrome X is a rather misleading and unhelpful term that describes patients with chest pain, angiographically normal coronary arteries and ST segment depression with exercise. The supposition is that the ST segment change represents myocardial ischaemia (rather than a false positive response) and that pain is due to myocardial ischaemia. It is quite reasonable to suppose that some patients have small vessel abnormalities that might give rise to myocardial ischaemia, and there are data to support this concept, but it is also quite probable that many patients with this diagnostic label have non-cardiac pain and a false positive exercise test.

The term 'syndrome X' does little to help the patient and is made more confusing by the coexistence of another (metabolic) syndrome X, also known as the insulin resistance syndrome. Furthermore, there appears to be an overlap between the two groups, since some patients with cardiac syndrome X also have insulin resistance[7].

Microvascular angina is perhaps a more useful term, not only indicating the site of pathology but also obviating the need for exercise test criteria within the definition. Some years ago it was shown that a proportion of patients with chest pain and angiographically normal coronary arteries have impaired coronary flow reserve, pointing to a microvascular abnormality that might give rise to ischaemia and chest pain.

In routine clinical practice, if a patient with troublesome chest pain is found to have normal coronary arteries, a sensible approach would be to reassure the patient (since prognosis is excellent in this patient group), exclude obvious musculoskeletal causes, and to try empirical treatment with a proton pump inhibitor. If symptom relief remains troublesome then a formal gastroenterological opinion would be reasonable. If the patient truly derives symptom relief with vasodilators (calcium antagonists, nitrates) then it is reasonable to continue this treatment, but the patient should be informed quite clearly that she does not have 'angina' in its usual sense.

7. How useful is history taking for establishing the cause of chest pain in women?

Establishing the cause of chest pain in women based on history alone is extremely difficult[8]. The nature of the chest pain is less predictive in women. Up to a third of women with 'typical' angina have no evidence of coronary artery disease at subsequent coronary angiography. In contrast, over 90% of men with typical angina have established coronary artery disease. The less typical the history, the more difficult the situation becomes. Consequently, the diagnosis should not be based on history alone.

8. What is the role of treadmill testing in women with chest pain?

Although treadmill exercise testing is non-invasive, readily available and relatively cheap, it has its limitations. False positive exercise tests are more common in women whereas false negative tests are more common in men. Younger women with few or no risk factors are unlikely to have coronary artery disease and are therefore more likely to have a false positive exercise test, making interpretation of the exercise test result difficult. Exercise testing can be misleading in up to a third of cases overall, but is a more valuable diagnostic tool in women with more typical symptoms and a worse risk factor profile[9]. However, it should be remembered that exercise testing not only gives information about ST segment response to exercise, but also symptom reproduction, exercise capacity, blood pressure response and the development of rhythm disturbance.

9. What are the alternatives to exercise testing and how should they be used?

Other forms of stress testing, such as stress echocardiography[10] and stress thallium scintigraphy[11] are more accurate than treadmill stress testing for assessing women with chest pain. However, they are less readily available, more labour-intensive and more expensive. They have a particular role in the assessment of women with a moderate, rather than low or high, risk of coronary artery disease. Younger women with atypical symptoms and minimal or no cardiovascular risk factors are at low risk of significant coronary artery disease. A typical history and an increasing number of cardiovascular risk factors lower the threshold for investigation (**Fig 12.1**). Coronary angiography remains the gold standard for establishing a diagnosis of coronary artery disease, although historically women are less likely to be referred for angiography and subsequent intervention. These differences may be explained by gender bias, age bias and a lower likelihood of coronary artery disease in women. With increasing awareness of the importance of heart disease it is hoped that women will be referred more appropriately for coronary angiography.

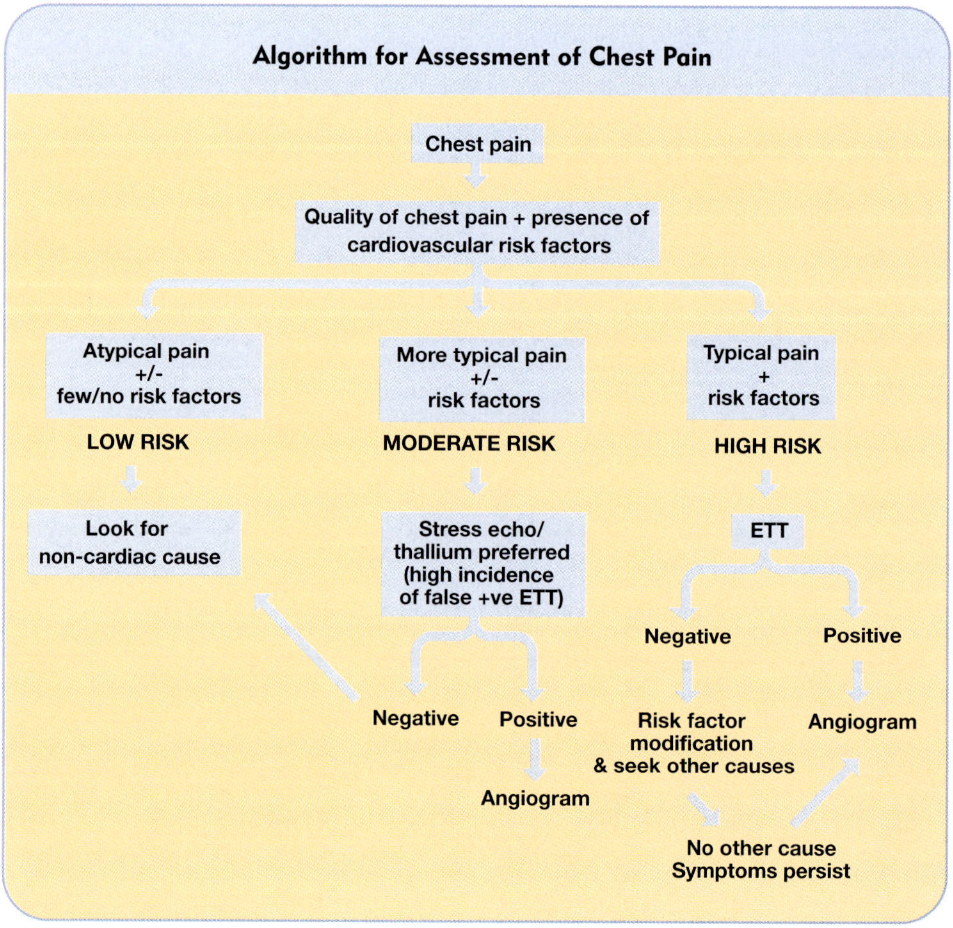

Fig. 12.1 Algorithm for assessment of chest pain. ETT, exercise tolerance test.

References

1. Holdright DR. Risk factors for cardiovascular disease in women. *J Hum Hypertens* 1998;**12**:667–73.
2. Hulley S, Grady D, Bush T, *et al*. for the Heart and Estrogen/progestin Replacement Study (HERS) Research Group. Randomized trial of estrogen plus progestin for secondary prevention of coronary heart disease in postmenopausal women. *J Am Med Assoc* 1998;**280**:605–13.
3. Delmas PD, Bjarnason NH, Mitlak BH, *et al*. Effects of raloxifene on bone mineral density, serum cholesterol concentrations, and uterine endometrium in postmenopausal women. *N Engl J Med* 1997;**337**:1641–7.
4. Murabito JM, Evans JC, Larson MG, *et al*. Prognosis after the onset of coronary heart disease. An investigation of differences in outcome between the sexes according to initial coronary disease presentation. *Circulation* 1993;**88**:2548–55.
5. Sullivan AK, Holdright DR, Wright CA , *et al*. Chest pain in women: clinical, investigative and prognostic features. *Br Med J* 1994;**308**:883–6.
6. Saltissi S. Cardio-oesophageal reflex and "linked angina" – is the way to a man's (or woman's) heart through the stomach? *Eur Heart J* 1996;**17**:329–31.
7. Botker HE, Moller N, Ovesen P, *et al*. Insulin resistance in microvascular angina (syndrome X). *Lancet* 1993;**342**:136–40.
8. Detry J-MR, Kapita BM, Cosyns J, *et al*. Diagnostic value of history and maximal exercise electrocardiography in men and women suspected of coronary heart disease. *Circulation* 1977;**56**:756–61.
9. Curzen N, Patel D, Clarke D, *et al*. Women with chest pain: is exercise testing worthwhile? *Heart* 1996;**76**:156–60.
10. Masini M, Picano E, Lattanzi F, *et al*. High dose dipyridamole-echocardiography test in women: correlation with exercise-electrocardiography test and coronary arteriography. *J Am Coll Cardiol* 1988;**12**:682–5.
11. Friedman TD, Greene AC, Iskandrian AS, *et al*. Exercise thallium-201 myocardial scintigraphy in women: correlation with coronary arteriography. *Am J Cardiol* 1982;**49**:1632–7.

13. The Elderly

Margot A Gosney

1. Is angina pectoris a common problem in the elderly?

The incidence of ischaemic heart disease increases with age. Although it is relatively uncommon under the age of 40 years, the frequency rises rapidly after this age in males and to a lesser extent in females. In older age groups the incidence is approximately equal in both males and females, and while the number of deaths in some countries and some age groups has fallen this is not the case in older patients in the UK[1]. Cardiovascular disease is the main cause of death in the UK with over 150 000 deaths in 1995[2]. In elderly people ischaemic heart disease is responsible for over one-half of all deaths and contributes to much of the disability that is seen in patients with heart failure. Angina as a manifestation of ischaemic heart disease is thus commonly seen in many older patients.

2. Are there problems when diagnosing angina pectoris in older people?

The original description by William Heberden in 1768 illustrated the four cardinal features of angina pectoris. That is its location (the retrosternal region) and radiation (particularly to the left arm), relationship to exertion, relatively short duration (described as 1–10 minutes) and strangling quality. The presence of 'textbook' angina pectoris ensures prompt diagnosis. However, silent ischaemia is particularly common in older people and results in incorrect or late diagnosis in up to 40% of cases.

3. What is the evidence for silent ischaemia in older people?

First, the evidence comes from exercise testing in both asymptomatic healthy elderly and those suspected of having silent ischaemia. An incidence of 36% in patients aged 70 years or older in whom silent ischaemia is suspected contrasts with an incidence of 15% in asymptomatic volunteers in their ninth decade. The second area of evidence is from histopathological verification of vessel disease at post mortem. While autopsy studies may lack some sensitivity, the finding of 72% of men and 54% of women aged 70 years or older to have 75% or greater stenosis of at least one major coronary artery suggests that this elderly group are often under-represented in epidemiological studies that rely solely on clinical diagnosis.

4. Why is silent ischaemia so common in older people?

The presence of other coexisting diseases such as pulmonary insufficiency, stroke or arthritis may ensure that the older person is less likely to exercise to a point of critical ischaemia. There is some evidence that the elderly have reduced sensitivity to pain and thus do not experience 'angina'. However, the evidence for this is conflicting and it may be more likely that this group of elderly subjects is more stoical in their approach to symptoms and thus less likely to present with 'textbook' angina.

5. How might the older patient with angina present?

In the absence of typical chest pain, symptoms such as dyspnoea or palpitations may suggest a cardiac origin. However, in some older people or those with a degree of mental impairment, angina may present atypically as one of the 'giants of geriatric medicine' such as confusion, incontinence, falls, or as a patient who has "gone off their legs".

6. Are the risk factors for the development of ischaemic heart disease the same in the elderly as in young subjects?

Hypertension, elevated lipids and smoking are all important risk factors in the development of ischaemic heart disease, and all are amenable to intervention with resultant reduction in both morbidity and mortality. Other factors such as physical activity, obesity and oestrogen status in women have an important role, although much evidence in elderly people is anecdotal[3,4].

7. What is the evidence of improved outcome due to the management of hypertension in older people?

Reduction in both systolic and diastolic blood pressure is efficacious in older patients. The treatment of isolated systolic hypertension (160 mmHg or more) in subjects aged 60 years or above reduces fatal or non-fatal stroke by 36%, and non-fatal myocardial infarction or coronary death by 27%, and results in an overall 32% reduction of all major cardiovascular events[5].

The treatment of diastolic hypertension also reduces both cardiac and stroke morbidity and mortality[6], although some evidence has shown that if diastolic pressure is reduced to below 85 mmHg there is a noticeable increase in both cardiac morbidity and mortality[7].

8. What is the evidence of improved outcome due to the management of lipids in older patients with ischaemic heart disease?

The evidence is twofold. First, in patients with elevated lipids and second in those with normal lipids. In the 4S study of subjects 60 years or above with an elevated cholesterol and a previous cardiac event the effect cholesterol lowering was a relative risk reduction to 0.71 of a major coronary event in the treated group[8]. Indeed the absolute risk reduction for both all cause and coronary heart disease mortality in the treated elderly subjects was approximately twice as great than in the younger treated group. The CARE trial, which studied patients 65–75 years of age with lipids in the average range who had a previous cardiac event and plasma total cholesterol of less than 6.2 mmol/l, showed that to prevent a major coronary event 11 patients would need to be treated for five years and to prevent a coronary death 22 patients would need to be treated for five years[9]. The trial concluded, therefore, that in older patients following a myocardial infarction and in the presence of a normal cholesterol level, lipid lowering provided cardiovascular protection.

9. What are the most likely comorbidities in angina pectoris in the elderly?

Heart failure commonly coexists with angina pectoris and its cause is often impaired myocardial contractility as a result of the ischaemic heart disease.

Although the presence of hypertension in patients with angina pectoris is not as common as the coexistence of heart failure, it is of increasing importance due to evidence that the treatment of lower levels of systolic blood pressure have increasing benefits to older patients.

10. How does one optimally treat angina in patients with hypertension?

The prevalence of coronary artery disease in patients with hypertension is high, and hypertension occurs in approximately 60% of patients with coronary artery disease. The management of hypertension is vital, particularly in elderly hypertensive men who have the highest incidence of ischaemic episodes. As with younger patients, nitrates, aspirin, calcium antagonists and, in selected cases, beta-blockers should be considered as mainstay therapy. All such drugs have a role in the management of angina, and beta-blockers are still considered by many to provide a therapeutic option for the management of hypertension in older subjects. Additionally some calcium antagonists have anti-hypertensive as well as anti-anginal properties and may be useful when both conditions coexist[10]. However, although the combination of a non-dihydropyridine calcium antagonist such as diltiazem or verapamil with a beta-blocker offers synergistic anti-ischaemic effects, the addition of their negative chronotropic action may lead to severe bradycardia, and thus in elderly patients may limit their usefulness[11].

11. How is angina in patients with heart failure optimally treated?

In the absence of any contraindications, all patients with systolic dysfunction should be treated with diuretics and an ACE inhibitor. In patients with predominantly diastolic dysfunction negative inotropic agents and ACE inhibitors are preferable to high-dose diuretics or vasodilators. ACE inhibitors that block the enhanced activity of the renin–angiotensin system and have vasodilator properties will treat the cardiac failure and have been shown to reduce the incidence of infarction, hospitalisation for cardiovascular disease and the need for coronary artery bypass surgery or angioplasty[12, 13]. As a result, the EUROPA trial is studying perindopril in stable coronary artery disease. It is suggested that ACE inhibition may improve endothelial function, exert anti-atherogenic and anti-proliferative activity, and also modulate sympathetic activity. Much of this evidence has arisen from the use of ACE inhibitors in the early and late phase of myocardial infarction, although their role in stable coronary artery disease has yet to be established.

There is some evidence for the use of non-selective beta-blockers in left ventricular dysfunction[14]. Carvedilol, a non-selective beta-blocker that also has alpha blockade and antioxidant effects, reduces both morbidity and mortality in patients with chronic heart failure[15]. The use of beta-blockers in elderly patients until recently has been discouraged. However, in the light of this evidence and in the presence of both angina and cardiac failure, the cautious introduction of such drugs should be considered.

References

1. De Bono DP, Hopkins A. The investigation and management of stable angina. Recommendations of a Working Party on the Joint Audit Committee of the British Cardiac Society (http://www.cardiac.org.uk/bcs).
2. Sivers F. Evidence-based strategies for secondary prevention of coronary heart disease, 2nd edn. Guildford: A&M Publishing, 1999.
3. Folson AR, Kaye SA, Sellers TA, *et al*. Body fat distribution and 5-year risk of death in older women. *J Am Med Assoc* 1993;**269**:483–7.
4. Paffenbarger RS, Hyde RT, Wing AL, *et al*. Physical activity, all-cause mortality, and longevity of college alumni. *N Engl J Med* 1986;**314**:605–13.
5. SHEP Cooperative Research Group. Prevention of stroke by antihypertensive drug treatment in older persons with isolated systolic hypertension. *J Am Med Assoc* 1991;**265**:3255–64.
6. Insua JT, Sacks HS, Lau T-S, *et al*. Drug treatment of hypertension in the elderly: a meta-analysis. *Ann Intern Med* 1994;**121**:355–62.
7. Cruickshank JM, Thorp JM, Zacharias FJ. Benefits and potential harm of lowering high blood pressure. *Lancet* 1987;**1(8533)**:581–4
8. Scandinavian Simvastatin Survival Study Group. Randomized trial of cholesterol lowering in 4444 patients with coronary heart disease: the Scandinavian Simvastatin Survival Study (4S). *Lancet* 1994;**344**:1383–9.
9. Lewis SJ, Moye LA, Sacks FM, *et al*. Effect of Pravastatin on cardiovascular events in older patients with myocardial infarction and cholesterol levels in the average range. Results of the Cholesterol and Recurrent Events (CARE) Trial. *Ann Intern Med* 1998;**129**:681–9.
10. Just H, Frey M, Zehender M. North of England evidence based guidelines development project: summary version of evidence based guidelines for the primary care management of stable angina. *Eur Heart J* 1996;**17(Suppl. G)**:20–4.
11. Spaulding C, Cabanes L, Weber S. The pharmacological and therapeutic basis for combined administration of beta blockers and calcium channel blockers in the treatment of stable chronic angina. *Br J Clin Pract* 1997;**88**:17–22.
12. Ferrari R. Effect of ACE inhibition on myocardial ischaemia. *Eur Heart J* 1998;**19(Suppl. J)**:30–5.
13. Garg R, Yusuf S. Overview of randomised trials of angiotensin-converting enzyme inhibitors on mortality and morbidity in patients with heart failure. Collaborative Group of ACE-Inhibitors Trials. *J Am Med Assoc* 1995; **273**:1450–6.
14. Cleland JGF, McGowan J, Clark A, *et al*. The evidence of betablockers in heart failure. *Br Med J* 1999;**318**:824–5.
15. Hansson L, Himmelmann A. Carvedilol in the treatment of hypertension – a review of the clinical database. *Scand Cardiovasc J Suppl* 1998;**47**:67–80.

14. Diabetics

Robert Kelly
Allan D Struthers

1. How common is coronary artery disease in diabetes?

Coronary artery disease affects 21% of IDDM (type 1) diabetics and 27–43% of NIDDM (type 2) diabetics[1]. This figure may in fact be higher with the newer classifications for diabetes[2]. Fifty-five per cent of diabetics die from cardiovascular disease[3]. In Framingham and the First National Health and Nutrition Studies (NAHANES), the risk of coronary artery disease was shown to be doubled in diabetics, especially in women, who are at a higher risk of mortality following their first myocardial infarction (MI). In NAHANES, diabetes accounted for 75% of male coronary artery disease mortality.

Silent infarction and ischaemia are also more prevalent in diabetics[4]. Total mortality is three times higher in diabetics[5], but ethnicity lowers the risk of heart disease in blacks and Afro-Caribbeans with diabetes. In the UKPDS study, 11% of newly diagnosed type 2 diabetics developed coronary artery disease (angina or MI) within eight years. In this study, 15% of men and 23% of women had ECG findings indicating myocardial ischaemia at the time of diagnosis. These type 2 diabetics are at a greater risk of mortality, which can be predicted from smoking, cholesterol (total cholesterol, LDL, HDL), hyperglycaemia and hypertension[6]. In fact, the presence of cardiac risk factors in addition to diabetes, increases the risk of cardiovascular mortality five-fold[3]. Twenty-five per cent of CABG and angioplasty patients are diabetic[7].

2. Is there a difference in cardiovascular risk between type 1 and type 2 diabetes?

In the majority of studies, no distinction is made between the two types of diabetes. With the longer duration of diabetes, coronary artery disease is the leading cause of death in type 1 diabetes. In type 2 diabetes, coronary disease is the leading cause of death independent of the duration of the disease[5].

In general, diabetics tend to have more diffuse and more distal coronary artery disease than non-diabetic angina patients. In those diabetics who infarct, there is a two-fold increased risk of acute mortality, reinfarction and late mortality[8]. This is further complicated by a five-fold increased risk of developing congestive heart failure compared with non-diabetics[5]. Cardiac death occurs more often in insulin-dependent diabetics. In type 2 diabetes, hypertension is more prevalent (45–60%), life expectancy is reduced, and there is excessive mortality across all age groups[5]. Hypertension added to diabetes increases the cardiovascular risk four-fold compared to nondiabetic normotensive patients[5]. Most diabetics are type 2 diabetics[9]. Their risk of mortality is four times greater than for type 1 patients. In addition to coronary disease, which is the most frequent cause of death in diabetics, stroke is four times more prevalent[5].

3. Is silent ischaemia more common in diabetes, and if so why and how important is this?

The patient with diabetes may have more severe coronary disease, but this may not lead to more angina because ischaemia may be silent and may only be discovered at exercise ECG testing or on myocardial perfusion scan. Naka *et al*. reported no difference in the number of positive exercise tests between diabetic and non-diabetic patients, but in diabetics with positive exercise tests there was 2.2 times more silent ischaemia than in controls ($P < 0.05$)[10]. In patients taking insulin or in those complicated by retinopathy, there is a greater risk of having silent ischaemia.

The Coronary Artery Surgery Study reported that diabetic patients with >70% stenosis of a coronary artery who had silent ischaemia, had a higher mortality than non-diabetic patients with silent ischaemia (59% 6-year survival vs. 82%; $P < 0.001$). In the absence of silent ischaemia, the survival rates were equal for both diabetic and non-diabetic groups. Some of these patients were referred for coronary artery bypass grafting. Those with silent ischaemia showed a trend towards improved survival compared with those patients managed with medical therapy (85% 6-year survival vs. 52%; $P < 0.08$). The presence of left ventricular systolic dysfunction did not alter the survival advantage[11].

Silent ischaemia is important as it may be a marker of sudden cardiac death and myocardial infarction[4]. Autonomic neuropathy increases the incidence of arrhythmic deaths. Some studies report that 32–42% of diabetics experience silent infarctions compared with 6–15% in non-diabetics[4]. The same trend was evident in the Framingham data in men but not in women. The importance of this point is that impaired pain sensation in diabetics with ischaemic heart disease suggests that angina is a poor discriminating symptom. On exercise and thallium scanning there is a higher incidence of silent ischaemia in diabetics compared to non-diabetics, further suggesting that ischaemia in these patients may be missed by symptoms alone.

The cause of silent ischaemia may relate to autonomic dysfunction. Langer *et al*. have reported that silent ischaemia is more common in diabetics with evidence of cardiac autonomic neuropathy[12]. In this study, silent ischaemia was found in 10% of the study group. The Asymptomatic Cardiac Ischaemia Pilot study (ACIP) found no significant difference between the incidence of ischaemic episodes during 24-hour ambulatory ECG monitoring and exercise testing. However, the diabetic subgroup was small by comparison with the control population, so it is conceivable that a greater number of diabetic cases may have produced more silent ischaemia[4]. Recent studies have shown that silent ischaemia occurs in 19% of type 1 diabetics, and in 22% of type 2 diabetics, the frequency of episodes being the same in both types[13]. In some groups the five-year survival for patients with autonomic neuropathy is only 50%[4]. Cardiac autonomic neuropathy in type 1 diabetes is associated with increased mortality[14]. In type 2 diabetes abnormalities of cardiac parasympathetic function advance more rapidly than those of sympathetic dysfunction, and the former is a strong predictor of 10-year mortality[15].

4. Are conventional antianginal medications appropriate in treating diabetics?

Treating diabetic patients with angina should be aimed at relieving symptoms and improving prognosis (**Fig. 14.1**). Modification of risk factors, especially lipids, glycaemic control, diet, exercise, blood pressure and smoking cessation are essential. Therefore, conventional antianginal treatment is appropriate but certain factors need to be borne in mind.

Glycaemic control

Tight glycaemic control in type 1 diabetics reduces coronary artery disease and cardiac events by 40%[16]. Similarly, intravenous insulin-dextrose regimes at the time of MI, improve prognosis in type 2 diabetics (including patients with a previous history of ischaemic heart disease) with a 30% reduction in three-year mortality and 11% absolute reduction in mortality[17]. However, the role of glycaemic control in preventing vascular events remains controversial as is shown by primary prevention studies (UKPDS) and the small number of high-risk angina patients included in DIGAMI.

Aspirin

In the Antiplatelet Trialists Collaboration, secondary prevention with aspirin reduces vascular events in both diabetic and non-diabetic patients[18]. The recommended dose of aspirin for stable angina patients is 75 mg once daily. However in diabetes, there can be enhanced platelet turnover and a higher dose (300 mg) may be more effective at suppressing this, especially for diabetics with established atherosclerosis[19].

Lipid-lowering therapy

In the 4S study, the overall risk of cardiovascular deaths and events in diabetics was reduced by 55%, compared with 32% in non-diabetics[20]. In CARE, both diabetics and non-diabetics had 23–25% reduction in mortality risk[21]. LIPID showed similar results[21].

The choice of lipid-lowering agent is influenced by the lipid profile. The goal of treatment is to achieve total cholesterol <4.4 mmol/l, LDL <2.6 mmol/l and non-HDL cholesterol <3.4 mmol/l (especially in type 2 diabetics)[21]. In diabetic angina patients, diet and good glycaemic control are first line therapy, followed by statins.

Beta-blockers

In diabetes, beta-blockers have a cardioprotective effect in the secondary prevention of MI, and they improve prognosis in postinfarct diabetics, reducing mortality by 50% compared with diabetics not receiving the same treatment[22]. This benefit is similar in both type 1 and type 2 diabetics following MI. Additionally beta-blockers reduce silent ischaemia. However, in type 1 diabetes, symptoms of hypoglycaemia may be masked when taking beta-blockers. Cardioselective beta-blockers reduce this risk, and are effective for secondary prevention of ischaemic heart disease[23]. In type 2 diabetes, continued use of beta-blockers may impair glucose tolerance. In diabetics with hypertension, beta-blockers should be used for treating patients with angina or following infarction[24].

Calcium antagonists

Calcium antagonists (CA) are indicated for treating angina, especially if beta-blockers are intolerable/contraindicated. Nifedipine is metabolically neutral and in some cases may lessen insulin resistance[25]. Amlodipine reduces silent ischaemia[26].

Recent studies have linked CA to adverse cardiovascular events in hypertensive patients with diabetes. However there is a lack of data from which to draw conclusions of harm. On the basis of larger trials, it could be concluded that CA +/- ACEi is a rational therapeutic choice in patients with both hypertension and diabetes[27].

Nitrates

Nitrates improve ST changes on the ECG in silent ischaemia but tolerance may still be a problem. No mortality data are available for nitrate therapy in angina patients with diabetes.

Trimetazidine (Vasteral) in diabetic angina may be very useful as its myocardial cytoprotective role reduces the development of diabetic cardiopathies[28].

ACE inhibitors

ACE inhibitors reduce cardiac ischaemic events following MI (SAVE, SOLVD)[29,30]. As the risk of mortality in diabetes is 50% greater, the benefit of ACEi is likely to be twice as much. The results of the EUROPA study in patients with normal LV function are awaited[31].

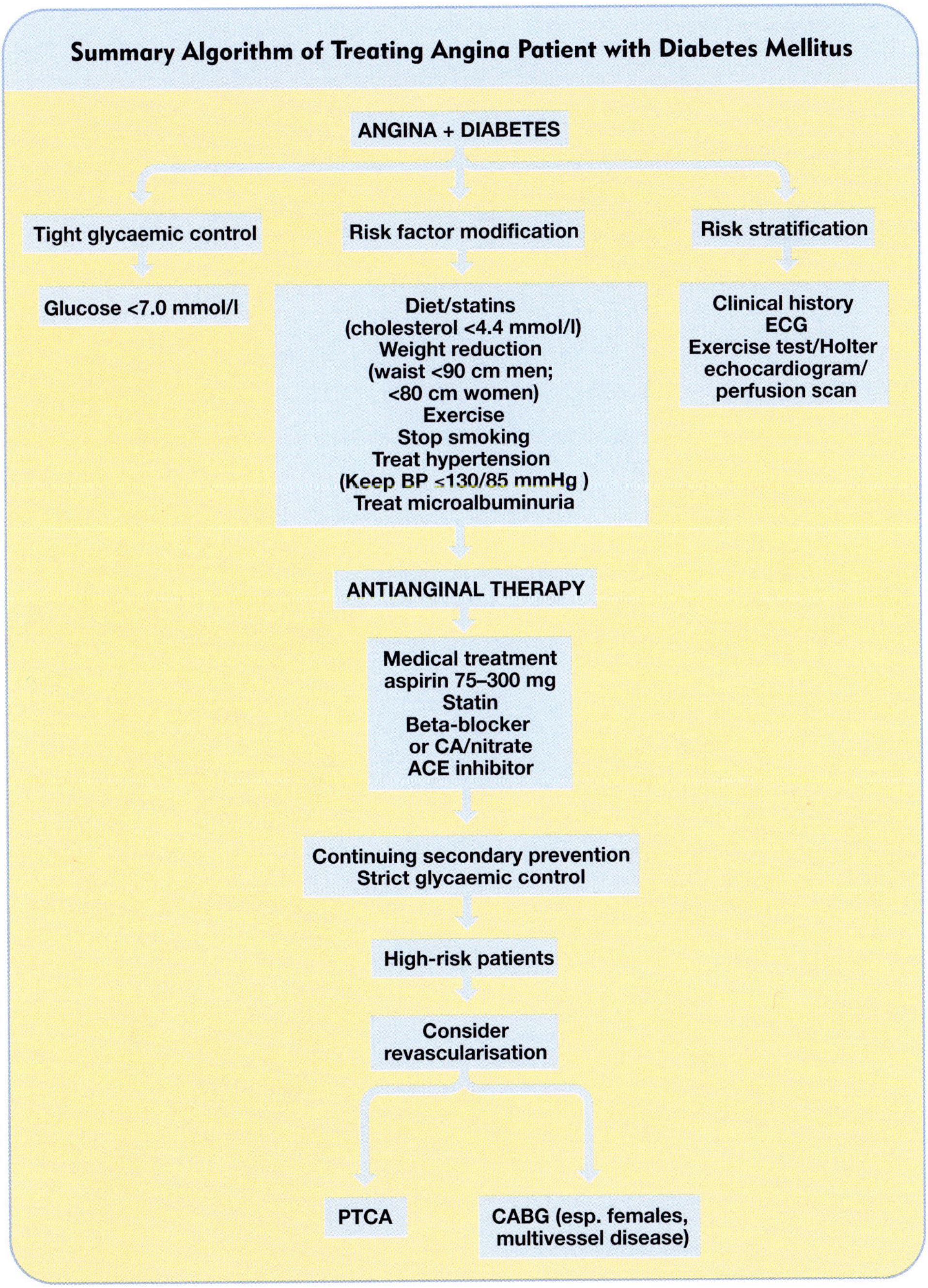

Fig. 14.1 Summary algorithm of treating angina patient with diabetes mellitus. Reproduced with kind permission of Lippincott, Williams and Wilkins[24].

Revascularisation

The most recent data suggests that CABG is superior to PTCA in diabetics, and that female diabetics with multi-vessel disease benefit most[32]. Diabetic patients who undergo angioplasty restenose four times more than non-diabetics, especially type 1 diabetics. Additionally they have significantly higher rates of MI, repeat revascularisation and overall mortality. Stenting improves the outcome[7]. CABG diabetics often develop more rapid progression of disease in both grafted and non-grafted native arteries and within vein grafts. Diabetes is a strong risk factor for late cardiovascular mortality after CABG[7].

5. Do oral hypoglycaemics increase the risk of cardiac death?

In one study, treatment with oral sulphonylurea drugs increased the rate of cardiovascular death, as compared with diet treatment only[33]. This could be because these agents prevent cardiac preconditioning and so worsen the effect of acute ischaemia in patients with chronic ischaemic heart disease. However, in UKPDS and Haffner's study[34], the use of oral sulphonylureas did not increase cardiac mortality in diabetic patients. But the UKPDS study excluded patients with current angina, yet 2% of patients had previous angina and 3% had previous MI. Further clarification of the 'cardiotoxic profile of sulphonylureas' in angina patients is needed. Glibenclamide on the other hand, improves survival in diabetics with angina, reduces arrhythmogenesis in MI, especially VF, and decreases the incidence of fatal MI[35]. An important point to note for angina patients with diabetes, is that metformin needs to be withheld prior to coronary angiography as it may exacerbate contrast-induced renal dysfunction.

6. How should obesity in the diabetic with heart disease be treated?

Weight reduction, reduced fatty-acid intake and increased physical exercise in type 2 diabetics improve metabolic control, reduce cardiovascular risk and progression of coronary artery disease, lower blood pressure and improve patient well-being and survival[5]. In type 1 diabetes, exercise reduces abdominal fat and improves lipid HDL profile, without adversely affecting hypoglycaemic episodes. Certain treatments, e.g. metformin, improve insulin sensitivity, reduce weight, improve lipid profiles and may benefit blood pressure and fibrinolysis[36]. Promising newer agents include the glitazones. However, troglitazone has been withdrawn in the UK due to hepatotoxicity[37].

An exciting development is the discovery of the protein tyrosine phosphatase-1B (PTP-1B) gene linked to hyperglycaemia and obesity in type 2 diabetes. The development of drugs to inhibit PTP-1B may help to overcome obesity in type 2 diabetes, though hypoglycaemia might be a problem[38]. Another promising area is the role of leptin secretion and its action in obesity, which may also lead to the development of drugs to treat obesity in type 2 diabetes[39].

References

1. Morrish NJ, Stevens LK, Fuller JH, *et al.* Incidence of macro-vascular disease in diabetes mellitus: the London cohort of the WHO Multinational Study of Vascular Disease in Diabetics. *Diabetalogia* 1991;**34**:584–9.
2. DECODE Study group, on behalf of the European Diabetes Epidemiology Study Group. Will new diagnostic criteria for diabetes mellitus change phenotype of patients with diabetes? Re-analysis of European epidemiological data. *Br Med J* 1998;**317**:371–5.
3. Stamler J, Vaccaro O, Neaton J, *et al.* Diabetes, other risk factors, and 12 year mortality for men screened in the Multiple Risk Factor Intervention Trial. *Diabetes Care* 1993;**16**:434–44.
4. Butler R, MacDonald T, Struthers AD, *et al.* The clinical implications of diabetic heart disease. *Eur Heart J* 1998;**19**:1617–27.
5. Scottish Intercollegiate Guidelines Network (SIGN). Management of diabetic cardiovascular disease. SIGN secretariat. Edinburgh: Royal College of Physicians, August 1997.
6. Turner RC, Millns H, Neil A, *et al.* Risk factors for coronary artery disease in non-insulin dependent diabetes mellitus: United Kingdom prospective diabetes study (UKPDS:23). *Br Med J* 1998;**316**:823–8.
7. Ellis SG, Narins MD. Problem of angioplasty in diabetics. Editorial. *Circulation* 1997;**96**:1707–10.
8. Malmberg K, Ryden L, Efendic S, *et al.* Randomized trial of insulin-glucose infusion followed by subcutaneous insulin treatment in diabetic patients with acute myocardial infarction (DIGAMI): effects on mortality at 1 year. *J Am Coll Cardiol* 1995;**26**:57–65.

9. Harris MI, Hadden WC, Knowler WC, *et al.* Prevalence of diabetes and impaired glucose tolerance and plasma glucose levels in US population aged 20–74 years. *Diabetes* 1987;**36**:523–34.
10. Naka M, Hiramatsu K, Aizawa T, *et al.* Silent myocardial ischaemia in non-insulin dependent diabetes mellitus as judged by treadmill exercise testing and coronary angiography. *Am Heart J* 1992;**123**:46–52.
11. Weiner DA, Ryan TJ, Parsons L, *et al.* Significance of silent myocardial ischaemia during exercise testing in patients with diabetes mellitus: A report from the Coronary Artery Surgery Study (CASS) Registry. *Am J Cardiol* 1991;**68**:729–34.
12. Langer A, Freeman M, Josse R, *et al.* Detection of silent ischaemia in patients with diabetes mellitus. *Am J Cardiol* 1991;**67**:1073–8.
13. Negrusz M, Moszczynska J, Zythiewicz D, *et al.* Frequency of silent ischaemic heart disease in patients with diabetes mellitus. *Pol-Merkuriusz-Lek* 1997;**3(14)**:53–6.
14. Sampson MJ, Wilson S, Karagiannis P, *et al.* Progression of diabetic autonomic neuropathy over a decade in insulin-dependent diabetics. *Q J Med* 1990;**278**:635–46.
15. Toyry JP, Niskanen LK, Mantysaari MJ, *et al.* Occurrence, predictors and clinical significance of autonomic neuropathy in NIDDM. *Diabetes* 1996;**45**:308–15.
16. The Diabetes Control and Complications Trial Research Group. Effect of diabetes management on macrovascular events and risk factors in the diabetes control and complications trial. *Am J Cardiol* 1995;**75**:894–903.
17. Malmberg K for the DIGAMI study group. Prospective randomised study of intensive insulin treatment on long term survival after acute myocardial infarction in patients with diabetes mellitus. *Br Med J* 1997;**314**:1512–15.
18. Antiplatelets Trialists' Collaboration overview of randomised trials of antiplatelet therapy. I: Prevention of death, myocardial infarction, and stroke by prolonged antiplatelet therapy in various categories of patients. *Br Med J* 1994;**308**:81–106.
19. Colwell J. Aspirin therapy in diabetes. *Diabetes Care* 1997;**20**:1767–71.
20. Pyorala K, Pederson TR, Kjekshus J, *et al.* The Scandinavian Simvastatin Survival Study (4S) Group. Cholesterol lowering with Simvastatin improves prognosis of diabetic patients with coronary artery disease: a subgroup analysis of the 4S study. *Diabetes Care* 1997;**20**:614–20.
21. Garg A. Treatment of diabetic dyslipidaemia. *Am J Cardiol* 1998;**81(4A)**:47B–51B.
22. Malmberg K, Herlitz J, Hjalmarson A, *et al.* Effects of metoprolol on mortality and late infarction in diabetics with suspected acute myocardial infarction. Retrospective data from two large studies. *Eur Heart J* 1989;**10**:423–8.
23. Rehnquist N, Hjemdahl P, Biling E, *et al.* Effects of Metoprolol vs Verapamil in patients with stable angina pectoris. The Angina Prognosis study in Stockholm (APSIS). *Eur Heart J* 1996;**17**:76 81.
24. The National High Blood Pressure Education Program Working Group. National High Blood Pressure Education Programme Working Group Report on Hypertension in Diabetes. *Hypertension* 1994;**23**:145–58.
25. Opie LH, Frishman WH, Thadani U. Chapter 3: Calcium channel antagonists. *Drugs in Cardiology*, 4th edn. London: WB Saunders Company, 1995:50–82.
26. Litchlen PR, Fisher LD. Analysis of arrhythmias in the Circadian Antiischaemia Program in Europe (CAPE). *J Cardiovasc Pharmacol* 1999;**33**:135–9.
27. Parving H-H. Calcium antagonists and cardiovascular risk in diabetes. *Am J Cardiol* 1998;**82**:42R–44R.
28. Pogatsa G. New concepts in the treatment of diabetic cardiopathies. *Orv-Hetil* 1997;**138**:1491–4.
29. Moye LA, Pfeffer MA, Wun CC, *et al.* Uniformity of captopril benefit in the SAVE Study: subgroup analysis. Survival and Ventricular Enlargement Study. *Eur Heart J* 1994;**15(Suppl. B)**:28.
30. Shindler DM, Kostis JB, Yusuf S, *et al.* SOLVD investigators. Diabetes mellitus a predictor of morbidity and mortality in the studies of left ventricular dysfunction (SOLVD) trials and registry. *Am J Cardiol* 1996;**77**:1017–20.
31. Simoons ML, Vos J, deFeyter PJ, *et al.* EUROPA substudies of pathophysiological concepts. European trial on reduction of cardiac events with perindopril in stable coronary artery disease. *Eur Heart J* 1998;**19(Suppl. J)**:J56–60.
32. Jacobs AK, Kelsey SF, Brooks M, *et al.* Better outcome for women compared to men undergoing coronary revascularization: a report from the bypass angioplasty revascularization investigation (BARI). *Circulation* 1998;**98**:1279–85.
33. University Group Diabetes Programme. A study of the effects of hypoglycaemic agents on vascular complications of patients with adult onset diabetes. *Diabetes* 1976;**25**:1129–53.
34. Haffner SM, Lehto S, Ronnemaa T, *et al.* Mortality from coronary artery disease in subjects with type 2 diabetes and in nondiabetic subjects with and without prior myocardial infarction. *N Eng J Med* 1998;**339**:229–34. *Comments* **339**:1714–16.
35. Pogatsa G. What kind of cardiovascular alterations could be influenced positively by oral antidiabetic agents? *Diabetes Res Clin Pract* 1996;**31**:S27–31.
36. Palumbo PJ. Metformin: effects on cardiovascular risk factors in patients with non-insulin dependent diabetes mellitus. *J Diabetes Complications* 1998;**12**:110–19.
37. Wise J. Diabetes drug withdrawn after reports of hepatic events. *Br Med J* 1997;**315**:1559–64.
38. Josefson D. Scientists discover a gene involved in diabetes and obesity. *Br Med J* 1999;**318**:689a.
39. O'Rahilly S, Savill J. Science, medicine, and the future: Non-insulin dependent diabetes mellitus: the gathering storm. *Br Med J* 1997;**314**:955–65.

15. Uncontrolled Chronic Angina

Michael Chester
Clare Hammond
Austin Leach

1. What is chronic refractory angina?

When Heberden coined the term 'angina pectoris' in the middle of the 18th century it was merely a phrase that accurately conveyed the symptoms described by patients[1]. Since then the term has become so intimately associated with myocardial ischaemia that for many clinicians angina pectoris *means* myocardial ischaemia.

Angina is a major disabling, chronic pain condition and treatment is based on the anti-ischaemia model. This approach is highly effective for most angina sufferers, the majority of whom respond to behavioural changes and simple medication. Where these treatments fail, sufferers require more invasive therapies such as angioplasty or coronary artery bypass surgery. Over the past few years there have been tremendous advances that have allowed surgeons and cardiologists to treat ever more complex and technically difficult coronary disease more effectively. Unfortunately for a growing number of patients with advanced coronary disease a point is reached when neither anti-anginal medication nor revascularisation can alleviate the angina.

Terminology

Several different terms are in use to describe this condition: intractable angina, end-stage angina, resistant angina and refractory angina. In order to avoid the confusion generated by this the following definition has been adopted by the UK National Refractory Angina Guideline group (see below).

Refractory angina is a clinical diagnosis. It is based on the presence of symptoms of angina that are thought to be caused by ischaemia due to advanced coronary disease and which are not controllable by a combination of maximal anti-anginal medication, angioplasty or coronary artery bypass surgery.

The presence of demonstrable myocardial ischaemia is desirable but is not an absolute requirement for including a patient in the guideline process. As the patient moves through successive stages of the treatment algorithm it becomes increasingly important that ischaemia is confirmed, especially when high-risk, high-cost procedures are considered. The choice of investigation must be at the discretion of the individual clinician, considering local expertise and availability, and the level of confidence in the clinical diagnosis. A recent questionnaire circulated to consultant cardiologists in the UK revealed that the vast majority of respondents support this proposal.

2. What is the aim of treatment in refractory angina pectoris?

Once the major risk factors (raised cholesterol, hypertension and smoking) have been addressed, no treatment has been shown to improve the refractory angina sufferer's prognosis. Thus the primary aim of therapy is to improve the patient's quality of life by ameliorating the effects of angina. The clinician must balance the beneficial effects of therapy against the negative impact of the side effects. The most widely recognised clinical example of this in angina management is the use of beta-blocking agents that famously impair erectile function in a way that detracts from their beneficial effects on angina. This approach is even more critical when therapies that involve high risk and irreversible adverse effects are under consideration.

3. What is the starting point?

Diagnosis

The diagnosis of refractory angina pectoris is a clinical one and regular angiographic review is required to exclude revascularisable disease. The label 'unrevascularisable' does not necessarily mean that the patient has such severe diffuse distal vessel disease that revascularisation will never be an option. In fact, the majority of patients usually have a combination of unrevascularisable disease affecting one area and relatively good flow through good grafts or native vessels supplying another. A sudden deterioration in symptoms should raise suspicions that new 'revascularisable' disease might have developed.

The patient-centred management model

The starting point to refractory angina pectoris management is to adopt a patient-centred management model in which the clinician concentrates on determining which treatments are the most likely to fulfil the patient's objectives. As with all (complex) medical conditions, a good working relationship between the clinician and the patient is essential. This is based on mutual respect and understanding. Problems and beliefs that have evolved over many years of conventional therapy cannot be dealt with in a short time. In addition, many of the treatments used in refractory angina pectoris management are counter-intuitive to the veteran patient entrained in the ischaemia-centred model of angina management. A great deal of patience is required to help patients and their families understand the basis for the recommendations that 'do not make sense' according to their understanding of angina.

Treatment contract

All too often a clear description of angina pectoris triggers a reflex diagnostic then therapeutic process that only tackles the patient's concerns indirectly. Disappointment inevitably results when expectation is not matched by outcome and is avoidable if care is taken to ensure that all concerned (the patient, their carers and the doctor) have realistic expectations. Extra clinic time must be set aside to facilitate a clearer understanding of what it is the patient really wants and in every case reach an agreement about what is realistic and achievable. At this stage it is important to appreciate that it is the effect that symptoms have on the patient's quality of life rather than the pain itself that matters. For example we have a number of patients whose angina improved following coronary artery bypass surgery but whose quality of life was severely restricted by their families' insistence that they should do nothing to provoke an 'attack'. Once the carers' concerns were addressed *THEN* the patient was able to lead a normal life. For others, especially young patients, even trivial angina is the equivalent of a 'ticking time bomb' which understandably produces disabling anxiety and eventually depression.

4. What is maximal anti-anginal therapy?

Anti-anginal therapy is designed to improve symptoms through reducing ischaemia. Clear explanation of the aims of therapy can be helpful in improving patient compliance. There is a false assumption that poor patient compliance is not a problem in painful conditions. Several groups of drugs are available and by the time a patient fulfils the criteria for refractory angina pectoris all classes in combination should have been considered. Thus most patients with refractory angina pectoris are receiving or have tried short-acting nitrates, long-acting nitrates, beta-blockers, calcium channel blockers and potassium channel openers. Newer agents such as trimetazidine, which has beneficial effects on symptoms independently of haemodynamic effects, may have a role in chronic refractory angina pectoris. Opioids can be useful and are included in the management algorithm.

5. What are the treatment options when oral therapy fails?

There are several non-revascularisation treatment options available for the management of refractory angina. These treatments vary enormously in terms of cost, safety and efficacy. However there is a dearth of comparative research studies and aside from a small placebo controlled trial of stellate ganglion blockade in 1965 none of the currently used therapies has been assessed in a placebo-controlled study. The National Refractory Angina Guideline group, using a modified Delphi method, has recently produced a provisional consensus view of best practice, which has been endorsed by the British Cardiovascular Interventional Society (BCIS). The group has been commissioned by the British Cardiac Society to submit the final guideline in 2000.

Best management stepwise algorithm for patients suffering from chronic refractory angina

The guideline group authors stress that it is a provisional guideline and that individual practitioners will have to take account of local resource provision. The guideline will be updated regularly, as new information on current therapies or new therapies becomes available, e.g. external counterpulsation.

1. Diagnosis

(a) Requires a cardiological and cardiothoracic surgical opinion that the patient has angina of ischaemic origin and that revascularisation is unfeasible. Regular angiographic review is recommended to exclude the development of 'new' revascularisable disease.

(b) Out-patient assessment to include: review of pain history, drug history and physical exam. It is essential to ensure that the patient has failed to respond to optimal medication. Poor compliance should be considered and the need for compliance explained. Simplification of the drug regimen is recommended.

(c) Exclude non-cardiac causes, e.g. costochondritis, intercostal neuralgia, anaemia, thyrotoxicosis, reflux oesophagitis (consider trial of proton pump inhibitors).

(d) It is important to consider the possibility that depressive disease may contribute a significant component to the patient's total pain experience. The Hospital Anxiety and Depression questionnaire is a simple screening tool that can help to identify patients who might benefit from psychiatric or psychological assessment. Note cardiac patients have high anxiety scores.

2. Out-patient counselling to include explanation of management plan, lifestyle advice (diet, smoking, physical activity). A realistic and achievable 'treatment contract' should be decided on so that the patient, their family and the clinical treatment team have an agreed objective.

3. Rehabilitation[2–8]. Based on recommended guidelines[9]: involving exercise programme, lifestyle advice, relaxation training.

4. Multi-disciplinary cognitive–behavioural pain management programme[10,11]. If appropriate, base on established psychological assessment methods, e.g. Hospital Anxiety and Depression score. A psychological assessment can be of value especially in determining whether formal psychotherapy may be of value.
5. Transcutaneous electrical nerve stimulation[12–14](**Fig. 15.1**).
6. Temporary sympathectomy. Stellate ganglion block[15–18], T3/4 paravertebral block in stages[19]. High thoracic epidural[20]. (See **Figs 15.2** & **15.3**.)
7. Spinal cord stimulation[21–28]. Implant data and outcome should be recorded in a registry (see **Fig 15.4**).

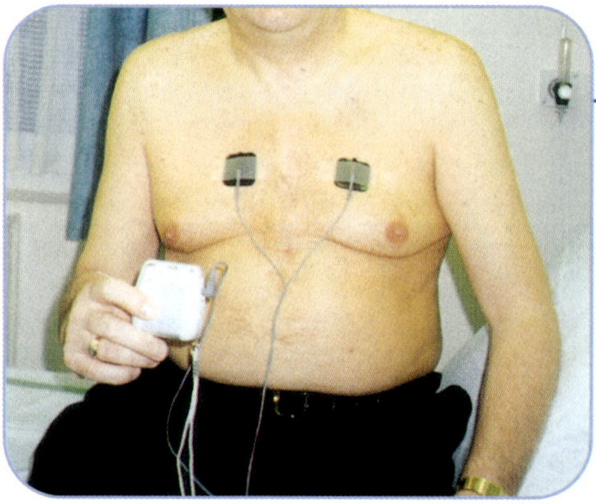

Fig. 15.1
Transcutaneous electrical nerve stimulation (TENS) with pads placed across the area of pain. It is recommended that the patient stimulates for one hour three times a day and when required. The position of the pads should vary to avoid skin irritation.

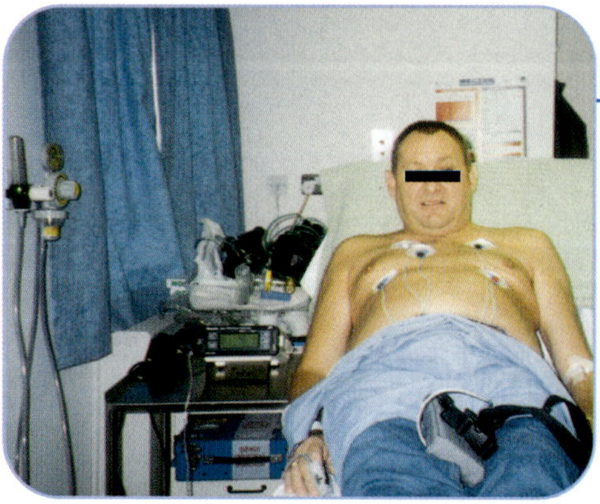

Fig. 15.2
The very low risks associated with sympathetic ganglion blockade[18] should be minimised by performing the blocks in an appropriate treatment area with full resuscitation facilities available. In the Cardiothoracic Centre, Liverpool, all procedures are carried out with at least two experienced operators in attendance.

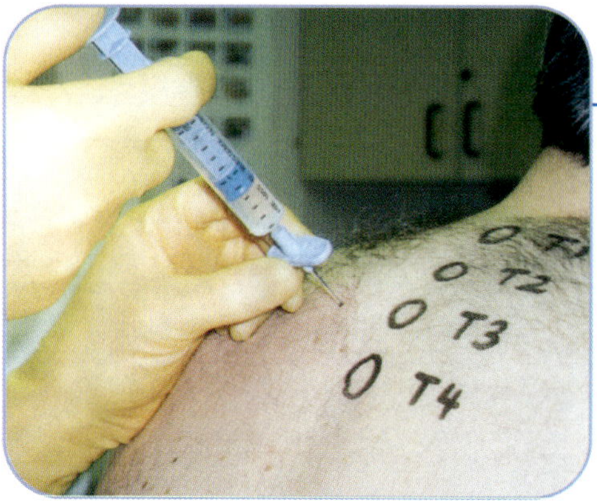

Fig. 15.3
Loss of resistance technique to locate paravertebral space at T3.

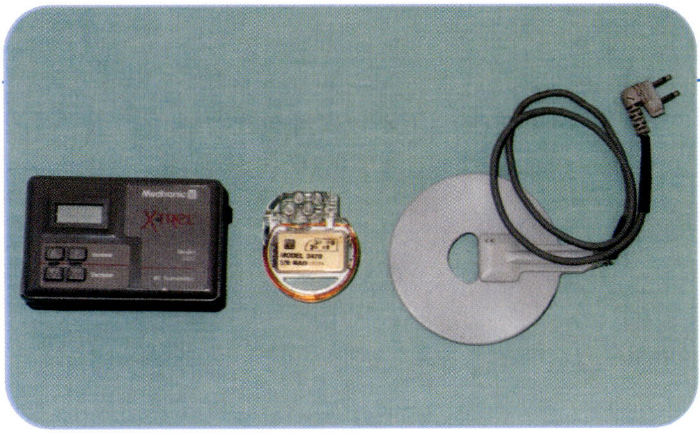

Fig 15.4
Xtrel spinal cord stimulation system with radiofrequency generator worn on the patients belt, implantable pulse generator and transmitter that is placed over the impulse generator. Reproduced with kind permission of Medtronic Ltd.

8. Opioids. There is limited evidence of the effectiveness of opioids in refractory angina. In clinical practice oral and transdermal opioids can be effective but can be limited by side-effects. Trial of epidural followed by intrathecal opioids might be beneficial[29].
9. Destructive sympathectomy[30–32]. Thoracoscopic, surgical, or phenol depending on local expertise.
10. Myocardial (percutaneous or transmyocardial) laser[33–41]. There is insufficient data to support this therapy outside clinical research. We recommend that these therapies should only be undertaken as part of a formal clinical trial.

Angina alone is not an indication for cardiac transplantation

A key recommendation of the guideline group is that closer links should be developed between the relevant practitioners, especially cardiologists and pain specialists.

CONCLUSIONS

Chronic angina that is refractory to medication and conventional revascularisation is a small but growing clinical problem. Several approaches are in use in treating these 'heart sink' patients and range from doing nothing, through to extremely low-cost and low-risk treatments and to high-cost and high-risk procedures. The UK refractory angina consensus guideline sets out a logical order in which these therapies should be tried based on the available evidence. These complex patients are best managed within a patient-centred multi-disciplinary framework with quality of life improvement as the primary aim of therapy. Treating these patients is highly rewarding if basic rules are applied: (a) aim to give the patient what he/she wants; (b) try the simplest and easiest therapies first.

References

1. Heberden W. Some account of a disorder of the breast. *Med Trans* 1772;**2**:9–67.
2. NHS Centre for Reviews and Dissemination, University of New York. Cardiac rehabilitation. *Eff Health Care Bull* 1988;**4**:1–2.
3. Horgan J, Bethell H, Carson P, *et al*. Working party report on cardiac rehabilitation. *Br Heart J* 1992;**67**:412–18.
4. Schuler G, Schlierf G, Wirth A, *et al*. Low fat diet and regular, supervised physical exercise in patients with symptomatic coronary artery disease: Reduction of stress-induced myocardial ischaemia. *Circulation* 1988;**77**:172–81.
5. Todd IC, Ballantyne D. Antianginal efficacy of exercise training: a comparison with beta blockade. *Br Heart J* 1990;**64**:14–19.
6. National Institute of Health. *NIH Consensus Statement, Physical Activity and Cardiovascular Health* 1995;**13(3)**:33.
7. Ornish D, Brown SE, Scherwitz LW, *et al*. Can lifestyle changes reverse coronary heart disease? *Lancet* 1990;**336**:129–33.

8. British Association for Cardiac Rehabilitation. In: Coats A, McGee H, Stokes H, *et al.* (eds). *Guidelines for Cardiac Rehabilitation*. Oxford: Blackwell Science, 1995.
9. Thompson DR, Bowman GS, Kitson AL, *et al.* Cardiac rehabilitation in the UK: Guidelines and audit standards. *Heart* 1996;**75**:89–93.
10. Lewin B, Cay EL, Todd I, *et al.* The angina management programme: A rehabilitation treatment. *Br J Cardiol* (in press).
11. Lewin B. The psychological and behavioural management of angina. *J Psychosom Res* 1997;**43**:453–62.
12. Mannheimer C, Carlsson C-A, Vedin A, *et al.* Transcutaneous electrical nerve stimulation (TENS) in angina pectoris. *Pain* 1986;**26**:291–300.
13. Borjesson M, Eriksson P, Dellborg M, *et al.* Transcutaneous electrical nerve stimulation in unstable angina pectoris. *Coron Artery Dis* 1997;**8**:843–50.
14. Mannheimer C, Carlsson C-A, Emanuelsson H, *et al.* The effects of transcutaneous electrical nerve stimulation in patients with severe angina pectoris. *Circulation* 1985;**71**:308–16.
15. Moore DC. *Stellate Ganglion Block*. Springfield: CC Thomas, 1954.
16. Wiener L, Cox JW. Influence of stellate ganglion blockade on angina pectoris and the post exercise electrocardiogram. *Am J Med Sci* 1966;**252**:289–95.
17. Hammond C, Leach AA, Chester MR. Temporary sympathectomy in refractory angina. *Heart* 1999;**81(Suppl.)**:56.
18. Wulf H, Maier CH. Complications of stellate ganglion blockade: results of a survey. *Anaesthetist* 1992;**41**:146–51.
19. Leach A. Old ideas, new applications. *Br J Anaesth* 1998;**81**:113–15.
20. Blomberg SG. Long-term home self-treatment with high thoracic epidural analgesia in patients with severe coronary artery disease. *Anesth Analg* 1994;**79**:413–21.
21. Murphy DF, Giles KE. Dorsal column stimulation for pain relief from intractable angina pectoris. *Pain* 1987;**28**:365–8.
22. DeJongste MJ, Haaksma J, Hautvast RW, *et al.* Effects of spinal cord stimulation on myocardial ischaemia during daily life in patients with severe coronary artery disease. A prospective ambulatory electrocardiographic study. *Br Heart J* 1994;**71**:413–18.
23. Sanderson JE, Brooksby P, Waterhouse D, *et al.* Epidural spinal electrical stimulation for severe angina: a study of its effect on symptoms, exercise tolerance and degree of ischaemia. *Eur Heart J* 1992;**13**:628–33.
24. Greco S, Auriti A, Fiume D, *et al.* Spinal cord stimulation for the treatment of refractory angina pectoris: a two year follow-up. *PACE* 1999;**22**:26–32.
25. Mannheimer C, Eliasson T, Augustinsson L-E, *et al.* Electrical stimulation versus coronary artery bypass surgery in severe angina pectoris. The ESBY study. *Circulation* 1998;**97**:1157–63.
26. Anderson C, Hole P, Oxhøj H. Does pain relief with spinal cord stimulation for angina conceal myocardial infarction? *Br Heart J* 1994;**71**:419–21.
27. Sanderson JE, Ibrahim B, Waterhouse D, *et al.* Spinal electrical stimulation for intractable angina – long term clinical outcome and safety. *Eur Heart J* 1994;**15**:810–14.
28. Jessurun GAJ, Ten Vaarwerk IAM, DeJongste MJL, *et al.* Sequelae of spinal cord stimulation for refractory angina pectoris. Reliability and safety profile of long-term clinical application. *Coron Artery Dis* 1997;**8**:33–8.
29. Segal R, Murali S, Tipton K. Treatment of chronic unstable angina pectoris: use of a totally implantable programmable device for continuous intrathecal infusion of opiates: case report. *Neurosurgery* 1996;**38**:385–8.
30. Swetlow GI. Paravertebral alcohol block in cardiac pain. *Am Heart J* 1926;**1**:393–412.
31. White JC, Bland EF. The surgical relief of severe angina pectoris. *Medicine* 1948;**27**:1–42.
32. Flowthow PG. Sympathectomy for cardiac decompensation and coronary disease. *Surgery* 1952;**32**:796–802
33. Mirhoseini M, Cayton MM. Revascularisation of the heart by laser. *J Microvasc Surg* 1981;**2**:253–60.
34. Horvath KA, Cohn LH, Cooley DA, *et al.* Transmyocardial laser revascularisation: results of a multi-centre transmyocardial laser revascularisation used as sole therapy for end-stage coronary artery disease. *J Thorac Cardiovasc Surg* 1997;**113**:645–54.
35. Cooley DA, Frazier OH, Kadipasaoglu KA, *et al.* Transmyocardial laser revascularisation: clinical experience with twelve-month follow-up. *J Thorac Cardiovasc Surg* 1996;**111**:791–9.
36. Krabatsch T, Tambeur L, Lieback E, *et al.* Transmyocardial laser revascularisation in the treatment of end-stage coronary artery disease. *Ann Thorac Cardiovasc Surg* 1998;**4**:64–71.
37. Nagele H, Stubbe HM, Nienaber C, *et al.* Results of transmyocardial laser revascularisation in non-revascularisable coronary artery disease after 3 years follow-up. *Eur Heart J* 1998;**19**:1525–30.
38. Allen KB, Dowling RD, Heimansohn DA, *et al.* Transmyocardial revascularisation utilising a holmium:YAG laser. *Eur J Cardiothorac Surg* 1998;**14**(Suppl. 1):S100–4.
39. Trehan N, Mishra Y, Mehta Y, *et al.* Transmyocardial laser as an adjunct to minimally invasive CABG for complete myocardial revascularisation. *Ann Thorac Surg* 1998;**66**:1113–18.
40. Diegeler A, Schneider J, Lauer B, *et al.* Transmyocardial laser revascularisation using the holmium: YAG laser for the treatment of end-stage coronary artery disease. *Eur J Cardiothorac Surg* 1998;**13**:392–7.
41. Schofield PM, Sharples LD, Caine N, *et al.* Transmyocardial laser revascularisation in patients with refractory angina: a randomised controlled trial. *Lancet* 1999;**353**:519–24.

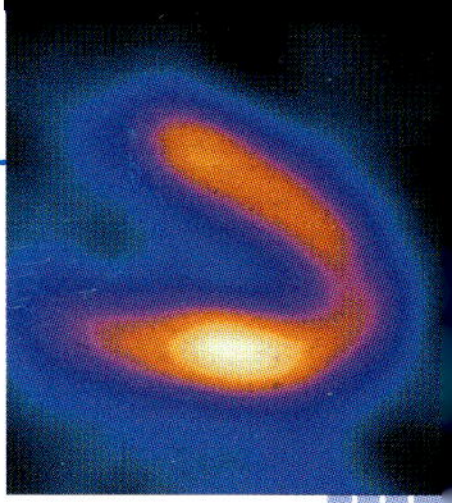

IV. Treatment Approaches

16. Treatment of Angina Pectoris

Henry Purcell
Sam Kaddoura

1. What are the goals of the treatment of angina?

The goals in treatment of angina are:

1. To improve prognosis by preventing myocardial infarction and death.
2. To minimise or abolish symptoms[1].

A general assessment of cardiovascular risk factors is essential (see Chapter 11). Particular emphasis needs to be placed on achieving 'normal' serum cholesterol levels and good blood pressure control. Similarly, it is important to reduce the risk of thrombosis with effective anti-platelet therapy.

2. What are the benefits of anti-platelet drugs?

There is now compelling evidence from randomised trials on the benefits of anti-platelet agents, principally aspirin, in the prevention of cardiovascular events in patients with established coronary heart disease (CHD)[2]. Aspirin in a dose of 75–325 mg/day reduces events such as non-fatal myocardial infarction (MI), non-fatal stroke or vascular death by about one-quarter. In the absence of contraindications, patients with stable angina and/or with previous MI, should be treated long-term with aspirin 75 mg/day [3].

3. What are the criteria for 'ideal' anti-anginal therapy?

Despite general guidelines, angina treatment needs to be individualised so that the most appropriate drugs are prescribed. Criteria for the 'ideal' anti-anginal are suggested in **Fig. 16.1**[1,4]. Unfortunately, no single drug yet fulfils all of these criteria.

4. What are the advantages and disadvantages of nitrates?

Organic nitrates have been used for the treatment of angina since the mid-1800s. Despite being available for such a long period, controversy still exists over whether the effects of nitrates are exerted primarily on the heart or on the peripheral circulation. It seems likely that multiple mechanisms are involved. Vasodilatation occurs through stimulation of cyclic guanosine monophosphate (cGMP) resulting in reduction of both pre- and afterload on the heart. Such

Criteria for the 'Ideal Anti-Anginal'

- **Efficacy: good symptomatic control as monotherapy**
- **Reduces overall cardiovascular risk – 'cardioprotective'**
  – anti-arrhythmic
- **Favourable quality of life/side-effect profile, e.g. does not cause headache, flushing, oedema, cold periphery, impotence, lethargy**
- **Acceptable to all patient groups, e.g. elderly, non-Caucasian patients**
- **Once-daily dosing and 24-hour anti-ischaemic activity**
- **Safe in combination**
- **Safe with concomitant disease**
- **Desirable adjunctive properties – antiplatelet activity**
  – fibrinolytic potential
- **Competitively priced**

Fig. 16.1 Criteria for the 'ideal anti-anginal'. Reproduced with kind permission of WB Saunders[1].

combined action results in diminished ventricular filling pressures, dimensions and wall tension and, ultimately, reduced energy needs. Nitrates also relax large coronary arteries and can reduce coronary spasm as well as enhancing coronary collateral flow, thereby redistributing flow from epicardial to subendocardial ischaemic territory. Although nitrates can cause a reflex increase in heart rate and contractility, such effects are usually not significant enough to negate their beneficial effects.

There are a variety of ways of administering glyceryl trinitrate (GTN) preparations. Short- and long-acting preparations are widely employed, and while sublingual tablets are rapidly effective for treating an acute attack, many patients find the spray more convenient. Also, because it is not exposed to air, the efficacy of GTN spray is maintained, thus removing the need to replace unused drug every few weeks. Angina sufferers should always carry one or other GTN preparation.

Sublingual nitrates improve exercise tolerance when taken prophylactically, but because the effects last a short time it is not possible to provide continuous prophylaxis. To circumvent this problem, a number of long-acting preparations have become available. However, this therapeutic approach is limited as nitrate tolerance, a phenomenon that appears to be dose- and time-dependent, soon develops[5], in some cases within 24–48 hours. Oral isosorbide dinitrate (ISDN) is similar to GTN but with a longer duration of action of two to three hours. It undergoes extensive 'first-pass' metabolism by the liver and its bioavailability is only about 25%, unlike its mononitrate (ISMN) metabolite which is 100% bioavailable. ISMN is usually taken two to three times a day, although once-daily sustained-release preparations can be used[6]; one recently introduced once-a-day ISMN preparation is combined with aspirin.

While all nitrates can induce tolerance, the transdermal GTN patch overcomes some of the disadvantages of the largely outmoded ointment that patients find messy to use. Because of more gradual absorption, the GTN patch may be particularly suitable for the patient who develops headaches with oral formulations. But the patch is expensive. Tolerance to continuous oral or transdermal nitrates develops rapidly and, in order to overcome this, nitrate-free intervals with patch removal at bedtime is recommended. The worry about intermittent nitrate therapy is that rebound exacerbation of symptoms may occur and that the patient may be unprotected in the early hours of the morning, when there is a well-documented increase in the incidence of myocardial ischaemia, myocardial infarction and sudden cardiac death[7]. Therefore, another class of anti-anginal agent, such as a long-acting beta-blocker or calcium antagonist, should be given in addition to nitrates.

Nitrates are safe. Side-effects include headache and occasionally postural hypotension. Only about 10% of patients are non-responders to nitrate therapy, and a further 10% experience side-effects requiring withdrawal of therapy. Although they do not have an intrinsic anti-arrhythmic action, nitrates may help to reduce mortality in the early phase of acute MI, but this has not been proven. A recent study has shown that ISDN effectively inhibits platelet adhesion and aggregation in patients with acute myocardial infarction who do not receive thrombolytic therapy.[8] These effects of nitrates may be of therapeutic and prognostic importance in this group of patients.

5. What are the advantages and disadvantages of beta-blockers?

Exertional angina may best be prevented using beta-blockers, and they tend to be used for prophylaxis rather than to alleviate the acute attack. Beta-blockers are indicated for most patients with more than the mildest angina[1]. They act predominantly by competitive inhibition of beta-receptors, of which there are two types, $beta_1$-receptors which are more prevalent in the heart, and $beta_2$, which are more common in the bronchi. Beta-blockers antagonise the effects of catecholamines to beta-receptors. Their principal anti-anginal actions are considered to be: slowing the heart rate at exercise and reducing cardiac output, thus reducing myocardial oxygen demand and increasing coronary blood flow through increased filling time in diastole. However, most also lower blood pressure, which conserves energy expenditure. The so-called cardioselective agents, i.e. drugs such as atenolol, preferentially bind to $beta_1$-receptors and are less likely to cause bronchoconstriction or Raynaud's-like side-effects, which are associated with $beta_2$-antagonism. However, cardioselectivity is a relative term, because at high doses $beta_2$-receptor blockade may occur. Beta-blockers are therefore best avoided in patients who may be susceptible to chronic obstructive airways disease.

A number of considerations must be made when choosing a beta-blocker. Agents that have intrinsic sympathomimetic activity (ISA), also called partial agonist activity (PAA), have less effect on resting heart rate and not only block beta-receptors but stimulate them depending on the prevailing level of sympathetic activity (**Fig. 16.2**). They may cause less bradycardia and offer advantages to patients with peripheral vascular disease, although such putative advantages are still a subject of some debate.

Beta-blockers are either lipid- or water-soluble (lipophilic or hydrophilic)[9], an effect that determines their duration of action and influences adverse effects. Lipophilic agents are well absorbed but undergo first-pass (hepatic) metabolism and produce variable plasma levels. They have short half-lives, and can pass the blood–brain barrier and therefore can cause central nervous system (CNS) side-effects such as nightmares. In contrast, hydrophilic agents are poorly absorbed, produce more uniform plasma levels and have long half-lives; their excretion is diminished in renal failure. They tend not to concentrate in the brain and therefore produce fewer CNS side-effects. The intermediate group of drugs undergo both renal and hepatic excretion.

Ancillary properties such as cardioselectivity, PAA and lipophilicity appear to be of little importance to their anti-anginal activity in patients with uncomplicated stable angina without evidence of airways disease. About 15–20%

Pharmacological Properties of Beta-Blockers

Drug	MSA	PAA	Cardioselective	Lipophilicity
Acebutolol	++	+	Yes	++
Atenolol	–	–	Yes	–
Betaxolol	++	–	Yes	++
Bisoprolol	–	–	Yes	+
Carvedilol[1]	++	–	No	++
Celiprolol	–	+[2]	Yes	–
Labetalol[1]	–	+?	No	+++
Metoprolol	–	–	Yes	++
Nadolol	–	–	No	+
Nebivolol	–	–	Yes	+++
Oxprenolol	+	+	No	++
Pinodolol	++	++	No	++
Propranolol	+++	–	No	+++
Sotalol	–	–	No	–
Timolol	–	–	No	++

MSA, membrane stabilising activity; PAA, Partial agonist activity; minus sign, none; [1]labetalol and carvedilol have additional $alpha_1$-blocking properties; [2]selective $beta_2$-agonist.

Fig. 16.2 Pharmacological properties of beta-blockers. Reproduced with kind permission of Martin Dunitz[9].

of patients will not tolerate long-term use of beta-blockers. The most common adverse effects include fatigue, dizziness, weakness, depression, and other CNS problems such as vivid dreams and insomnia. Care must be taken to observe the contra-indications to beta-blockers, such as heart block, asthma, etc., especially in patients with impaired left ventricular function, where heart failure may be precipitated. However, paradoxically, beta-blockers may benefit patients with mild to moderate heart failure[10]. Beta-blockers can adversely affect blood glucose levels and lipids, which may be of particular importance in the diabetic patient; some may also mask or prolong hypoglycaemia. However one retrospective study from the US suggests that beta blockers are associated with a lower mortality rate among elderly diabetic patients following myocardial infarction.[11] Other studies such as the United Kingdom Prospective Diabetes Study (UKPDS)[12] have also confirmed the efficacy of beta-blockade in reducing fatal and non-fatal events in diabetes. It should also be noted that sudden withdrawal of beta-blockers can occasionally result in rebound angina. Beta-blockers not only reduce anginal and ischaemic episodes, but may also exhibit antiarrhythmic activity. They may reduce the risk of ventricular fibrillation, and the risks of sudden death and reinfarction may be reduced in agents without PAA. Experimental studies suggest also that beta-blockers may have an antiatherosclerotic effect and prevent myocardial necrosis, but this has not been shown clinically.

6. What are the advantages and disadvantages of calcium antagonists?

Although calcium antagonists share the common property of inhibition of entry of calcium into the cell, resulting in vasodilatation of vascular smooth muscle and relaxation of myocardial muscle, they have quite distinctive pharmacological and haemodynamic properties (**Fig. 16.3**)[13]. Their anti-anginal effects appear to be mediated through a reduction of myocardial oxygen demand secondary to decreased afterload and myocardial contractility. All three classes – verapamil, diltiazem, and nifedipine – and their analogues, such as amlodipine, are effective anti-anginals. The nifedipine class (dihydropyridines) are potent vasodilators and cause the least depression of cardiac function; however, oedema, flushing and headache, which result from the vasodilator effects, may be troublesome in some patients.

Diltiazem may cause bradycardia; constipation and flushing are sometimes seen with verapamil, which can also cause significant depression of myocardial contractility, requiring caution in heart failure. These latter two agents may, however, be useful in suppression of supraventricular arrhythmias. The use of calcium antagonists in acute

Cardiovascular Effects of Amlodipine and Other Calcium Antagonists

	Amlodipine	Diltiazem	Verapamil
Heart rate	↔	↓	↓
AV node conduction	↔	↓	↓
Myocardial contractility	↔	↓↓	↓↓↓
Peripheral vasodilation	↑↑	↑	↑
Myocardial O_2 demand	↓	↓	↓

↑, increase; ↓, decrease; ↔, unchanged; AV, atrioventricular.

Fig. 16.3 Cardiovascular effects of amlodipine and other calcium antagonists. Authorised reprint from IJCP[13].

MI remains controversial, and they are perhaps best avoided in the acute phase of MI. Recent studies suggest that diltiazem may be beneficial following an uncomplicated MI in patients who do not have left ventricular dysfunction. Calcium antagonists are effective in the treatment of coronary spasm. They appear to cause few metabolic disturbances and seem to be 'lipid friendly'. Similarly they may be used in patients with peripheral vascular disease and diabetes. Although recent studies suggest that angiotensin converting enzyme (ACE) inhibitors may be more appropriate for the treatment of diabetic patients with hypertension, there is reassurance from further analysis of the Systolic Hypertension in Europe (Syst-Eur) trial[14], which showed that diabetics treated with the calcium antagonist, nitrendipine, had a significant reduction in cardiovascular mortality. But caution is needed when treating patients with heart failure. The only calcium antagonist licensed for treatment of angina and hypertension in heart failure is amlodipine.

The recently reported, Prospective Randomized Evaluation of the risk of the Vascular Effects of Norvasc Trial (PREVENT)[15] looked to see whether amlodipine would slow the progression of coronary atherosclerosis compared to placebo. While no benefit was demonstrated in terms of the primary outcome, angiographic change between the two groups of patients, the drug had a significant effect on a secondary measure, carotid atherosclerosis, measured by B-mode ultrasonography. Whereas the placebo group experienced a 0.033 mm increase in intimal–medial thickness (IMT) there was a 0.0126 mm decrease in the amlodipine treated group (P=0.007). There was no treatment difference in the rates of all-cause mortality or major cardiovascular events, although amlopidine use was associated with significantly fewer cases of unstable angina (**Fig. 16.4**) and coronary revascularisation. These beneficial effects have not been seen in previous angiographic trials with other dihydropyridine calcium antagonists such as nifedipine and nicardipine, in patients with stable coronary artery disease, even though these agents have proven anti-anginal efficacy, which suggests that amlodipine may have additional effects.

7. What are the advantages and disadvantages of potassium channel openers?

Nicorandil was the first potassium channel opener to be licensed for treatment of angina. It was initially developed in Japan, and it is now available in Europe. The compound consists of a nicotinamide vitamin group which acts as a potassium channel opener, and an organic nitrate. This provides a dual mechanism of action, where both preload and afterload are reduced producing a dose-related improvement in haemodynamics. Potassium channels, particularly those regulated by intracellular adenosine triphospate (ATP-sensitive) are ubiquitous in the heart and blood vessels, and are important modulators of cardiovascular function. On opening K_{ATP} channels, there is an increased efflux of potassium ions from the cell and the resting membrane potential is shifted towards more negative values (hyperpolarisation); this leads to an inhibition of calcium influx or indirect calcium antagonism, causing a fall in intracellular calcium concentration, relaxation of vascular smooth muscle cells and vasodilatation. Similarly to nitrates, nicorandil also leads to activation of the enzyme guanylate cyclase, which in turn induces an increase in intracellular cyclic guanosine monophospate (cGMP) and a decrease in intracellular calcium ions. Ultimately, this results in reduction in vascular tone, predominantly in the venous vascular bed, so that mainly the venous capacitance vessels are dilated. It is indicated for the prevention and long-term treatment of angina and has comparable anti-anginal efficacy to other standard anti-anginals[16] and does not appear to cause tolerance.

Nicorandil may possess 'cardioprotective' properties. In a number of models of ischaemia/reperfusion and myocardial stunning, and in canine models of coronary ligation, it may cause limitation of infarct size. It has also been show to prevent platelet aggregation. It has been suggested that nicorandil may mimic ischaemic preconditioning[17], a condition which appears to confer powerful protection against ischaemic necrosis. The clinical value of these appar-

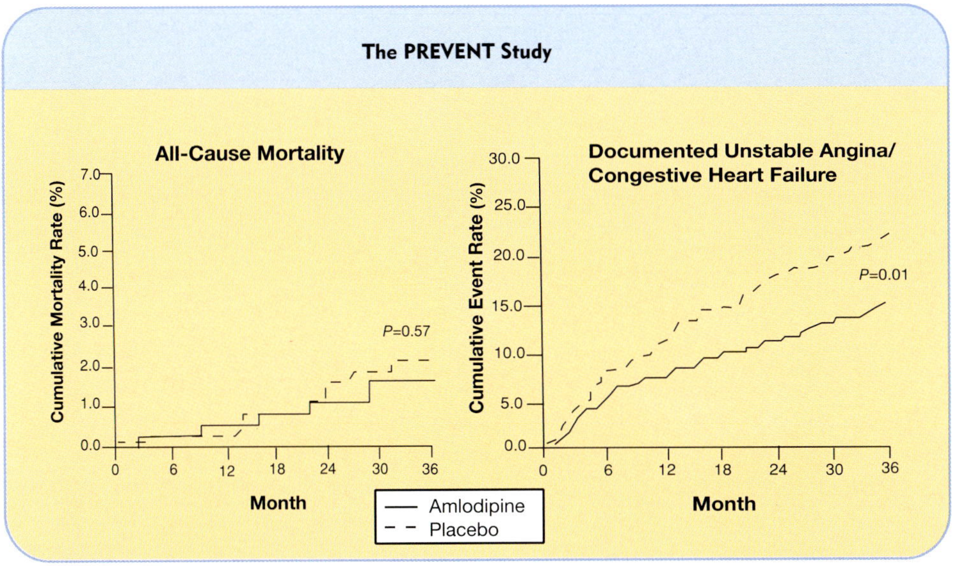

Fig. 16.4 Life-table curves for two prespecified event outcome measures in PREVENT. Reproduced with kind permission of Lippincott, Williams and Wilkins[15].

ent properties of nicorandil remain to be established. However, some preliminary studies suggest that nicorandil may provide additional anti-ischaemic effects in unstable angina patients who are already being treated with standard anti-anginals[18].

8. What are the advantages and disadvantages of cardioprotective metabolic modulators?

A number of metabolically active agents act to protect myocytes by optimising cardiac energy metabolism. These include trimetazidine and ranolazine, both piperazine derivatives, and the naturally occurring compound L-carnitine. Most clinical experience has been gleaned with trimetazidine which, although widely used throughout Europe, including the Republic of Ireland, is not currently licensed in the UK. Trimetazidine has anti-ischaemic properties which operate independently of any haemodynamic effects on heart rate, blood pressure (or rate pressure product) or myocardial contractility. It appears to act at the cellular level, maintaining creatine phosphate and adenosine triphosphate levels, and reducing cell acidosis, calcium overload and free radical damage[19]. During ischaemia trimetazidine shifts energy away from fatty acid metabolism towards glucose metabolism; it also decreases beta oxidation, which causes an accumulation of fatty acids and provides cell membrane protection by increasing phospholipid turnover.

CONCLUSIONS

No one anti-anginal drug has shown consistently greater efficacy in relieving chest pain or reducing exercise-induced ischaemia. In general, optimal doses of a given class of drug are preferable to routine use of combination therapy. Many patients respond to monotherapy when drugs are used at the appropriate doses; when monotherapy fails it is often advisable to add-in another class of anti-anginal medication. However, triple therapy, although widely used, is of doubtful benefit to the patient. Medical therapy, coronary angioplasty and coronary bypass graft surgery (see Chapter 17) must be considered together in an integrated approach to treatment.

References

1. Recommendations of the Task Force of the European Society of Cardiology. Management of stable angina pectoris. *Eur Heart J* 1997;**18**:394–413.
2. Recommendations of the Second Joint Task Force of European and other Societies on Coronary Prevention. Prevention of coronary heart disease in clinical practice. *Eur Heart J* 1998;**19**:1434–503.
3. Eccles M, Freemantle N, Mason J, and the North of England Aspirin Guideline Development Group. North of England evidence based guideline development project: guideline on the use of aspirin as secondary prophylaxis for vascular disease in primary care. *Br Med J* 1998;**316**:1303–9.
4. Purcell H, Mulcahy D. The search for the ideal anti-anginal agent. *MIMS* 1992;March **(Suppl.)**:1–3.
5. Rutherford JD. Nitrate tolerance in angina pectoris. How to avoid it. *Drugs* 1995;**49**:196–9.
6. Prakash A, Markham A. Long-acting isosorbide mononitrate. *Drugs* 1999;**57**:93–9.
7. Purcell H, Mulcahy D. Circadian rhythms and the onset of myocardial infarction:clinical implications. *J Cardiovasac Risk* 1995;**2**:510–14.
8. Gebalska, J, Wolk R, Ceremuzynski L. Isosorbide dinitrate inhibits platelet adhesion and aggregation in nonthrombolyzed patients with acute myocardial infection. *Clin Cardiol* 2000;**23**:837–41.
9. Purcell H, Mulcahy D. Management of angina pectoris and silent myocardial ischaemia. In: Elliott HL (ed.) *Current Issues in Cardiovascular Therapy*. London: Martin Dunitz, 1997.
10. CIBIS II Investigators and Committees. The Cardiac Insufficiency Bisoprolol Study II (CIBIS II): a randomised trial. *Lancet* 1998:**353**:9–13.
11. Chen J, Marciniak TA, Radford MJR, Wang Y, Krumholz HM. Beta-blocker therapy for secondary prevention of myocardial infarction in elderly diabetic patients. *J Am Coll Cardiol* 1999;**34**:1388–94.
12. UK Prospective Diabetes Research Group. Efficacy of atenolol and captopril in reducing risk of macrovascular complications in type 2 diabetes: UKPDS 39. *BMJ* 1998;**317**:713–20.
13. Purcell H, Waller DG, Fox K. Calcium antagonists in cardiovascular disease. *Br J Clin Prac.* 1989;**43**:369–79.
14. Staessen JA, Fagard R, Thijs L, *et al*. Randomised double-blind comparison of placebo and active treatment for older patients with isolated systolic hypertension. *Lancet* 1997;**350**:757–64.
15. Pitt B, Byington RP, Furberg CD, *et al*. Effect of amlodipine on the progression of atherosclerosis and the occurrence of clinical events. *Circulation* 2000;**102**:1503–10.
16. Purcell H, Fox K. Drugs in focus: nicorandil. *Presc J* 1999;**39**:39–43.
17. Kloner RA, Yellon D. Does ischemic preconditioning occur in patients? *J Am Coll Cardiol* 1994;**24**:1133–42.
18. Patel DJ, Purcell HJ, Fox KM. Cardioprotection by opening of the K(ATP) channel in unstable angina. Is this a clinical manifestation of myocardial preconditioning? Results of a randomized study with nicorandil. *Eur Heart J* 1999;**20**:51–7.
19. Jackson G. Angina, myocardial hibernation and trimetazidine. *Int J Clin Pract* 1997;**51**:347.

17. Percutaneous Transluminal Coronary Angioplasty and Coronary Artery Bypass Graft Surgery

Anu Garg

Roger Hall

Myocardial revascularisation is designed to augment coronary blood flow to areas of underperfused myocardium. Since the first coronary artery bypass graft (CABG) operation in 1964 and the first percutaneous transluminal coronary angioplasty (PTCA) in 1977, techniques, operator ability and equipment profile have improved considerably and are indispensable tools to the surgeon and cardiologist for managing patients with symptomatic coronary artery disease[1].

1. What are the indications for myocardial revascularisation?

Myocardial revascularisation is considered when angina pectoris is not controlled by medical therapy or when symptoms progress rapidly. In selected groups of patients these procedures can achieve a prognostic benefit as well. Cardiologists rely first on clinical grounds and then on the diagnostic coronary angiographic film before referring patients for PTCA and CABG[2].

PTCA

Recognised indications for PTCA +/- stent implantation include:

1. Discrete >50% stenosis in one or more major epicardial arteries.
2. Saphenous vein graft stenosis resulting in significant myocardial ischaemia.
3. Patients with persistent angina despite maximum medical treatment – targeting the 'culprit' lesion.
4. Acute myocardial infarction – where facilities and manpower are available PTCA is the gold standard treatment in these patients. Recanalisation of the occluded vessel and restoration of myocardial function is rapidly achieved with low rates of morbidity. Patients with contra-indications to standard thrombolytic therapy may be suitable for 'primary PTCA', particularly those in cardiogenic shock. 'Rescue PTCA' may be contemplated when thrombolytic therapy has not resolved objective evidence of myocardial ischaemia.

CABG

1. Left main coronary artery stenosis.
2. Left main stem coronary artery equivalent disease – ostial/proximal left anterior descending artery and left circumflex artery stenoses.
3. Multivessel coronary artery disease especially in those with impaired left ventricular function.
4. Redo CABG for severe coronary graft disease.
5. Immediately after failed PTCA – ongoing ischaemia or threatened occlusion with significant area of myocardium at risk or haemodynamic compromise (1% of PTCA).

2. What are the short- and long-term risks?

PTCA

The early risks of PTCA are low. The major complications include myocardial infarction 1.2–1.4%, emergency coronary artery bypass surgery 1.5–2.1%, and death 0.62–0.91%[3]. These events are usually the result of coronary arterial dissection and intracoronary thrombosis, which lead to vessel occlusion[4].

The major limitation to long-term event-free survival in those who have undergone successful PTCA is restenosis. This is defined as a >50% narrowing of the diameter of the lumen at the site of previously successful PTCA and occurs in about one-third of patients usually within six months after the procedure[5]. Restenosis is the result of the injury to the vessel leading to platelet aggregation, thrombus formation, inflammation and activation of smooth muscle cells. Most patients will present with recurrent symptoms of angina pectoris and myocardial infarction is rarely an initial manifestation of restenosis.

CABG

When coronary bypass surgery is undertaken on an elective basis and in the absence of recognised factors that increase the risks of surgery, mortality for coronary grafting is less than 1%. Complications can arise from anaesthesia, but the specific problems related to cardiopulmonary bypass include respiratory distress, renal impairment and a minor degree of neuropsychiatric abnormality, e.g. difficulty in concentration, memory loss and depression. These are usually transient. Major complications include:

1. Perioperative myocardial infarction – this is a cause of perioperative and early mortality. In surgery for stable angina this risk is 1.5–5% and doubles to nearly 10% in those operated on for unstable angina.
2. Stroke is reported to occur in 1%. This is the consequence of impaired cerebral perfusion during cardiopulmonary bypass[6].

The long-term risks of surgical revascularisation include stenoses developing in the graft and recurrent angina due to these or further disease in the native arteries. These problems are minimised by the use of arterial conduits (i.e. internal mammary artery) rather than saphenous vein grafts.

3. What is the role of intracoronary stents?

In the initial studies of PTCA, outcome results were affected by abrupt periprocedural closure of vessels (4–8%) and late restenosis (30–50%). Stents were developed to overcome these problems and in selected series of patients PTCA and stent insertion is as effective as CABG in relieving angina and is more effective than medical treatment alone[7]. Intracoronary stents are stainless steel alloy coils or tubes. They come in different angioplasty sizes (2.5–6 mm in diameter and 8–50 mm in length). They are premounted on a balloon and are expandable by balloon inflation. Using fluoroscopic screening of radio-opaque markers the stent is positioned across the stenotic lesion and deployed.

The use of stents has increased dramatically in the UK. Data from the British Cardiovascular Intervention Society show an exponential rise in the use of intracoronary stents from 2.7% of all procedures in 1992 to 45.9% in 1996[3] and 69% in 1998 (unpublished data). This is related in part to the complexity of coronary stenosis that is tackled by the interventionist and patients with coronary artery restenosis being referred for repeat procedures. The angiographic criteria for a lesion requiring stent insertion include:

1. Severe arterial dissection causing limitation of coronary blood flow.
2. Vessels with subtotal occlusion or complex plaques.
3. Long diseased segments.
4. Selected cases of graft disease.

Two important studies comparing conventional balloon angioplasty with stent implantation in single vessel coronary artery disease have shown that with intracoronary stenting fewer patients suffer myocardial infarction, stroke or require emergency CABG and repeat PTCA[8,9] in the months following the procedure. We await the results of ongoing randomised trials comparing coronary artery stenting with CABG in patients with multivessel coronary disease.

4. What are the complications related to intracoronary stents?

Although coronary artery stenting results in a larger post-procedure luminal diameter, the injury to the vessel can result in proliferation of neointimal matter that leads to restenosis within the stent. In-stent restenosis occurs in between 30 and 50% of patients (based on angiographic data) and subacute stent thrombosis in 0.8–3% of patients, usually within 7–10 days of the procedure. Antiplatelet treatment, particularly the synergistic combination of aspirin and ticlopidine, has reduced subacute stent occlusion from 5.4% (with warfarin) to 0.8%[4]. Clopidogrel is now used instead of ticlopidine as it has fewer side effects and seems to be as effective.

5. What risk factors increase the likelihood of complications with CABG?

The major predictors of mortality after CABG include[10–12]:

1. Urgency of operation – the more urgent the operation the worse the outcome.
2. Left ventricular ejection fraction – the more severely impaired the left ventricle, the greater the risk of surgery,
3. Severity of coronary artery disease, especially left main coronary artery stenosis.
4. Age – assuming age <65 years carries a relative risk of 1, for those aged 65–74 years the relative risk of CABG is 2.07, increaseing to 3.84 for those over 75 years of age.
5. Prior heart surgery – the relative risk is 3 compared to first-time CABG patients.
6. Sex – females have a greater reported relative risk than males (1.5–2.0). Reasons suggested include smaller body size, smaller diameter of coronary arteries and increased age at presentation.
7. Comorbidity – conditions include prior renal impairment, lung disease, neurological deficit (stroke) and peripheral vascular disease.

6. What have the trials comparing PTCA and CABG shown?

There have been several trials comparing PTCA and CABG. Differences such as patients with unstable and stable angina, those with single or multivessel disease and those enrolled in observational and randomised studies make interpretation of the results difficult. However, there do appear to be some consistent messages[13–15]:

1. Mortality after PTCA and CABG is not significantly different at 2–3 years. At five years, however, there is a slight survival advantage with CABG (95.1 vs 92% in those allocated to PTCA). This difference is mainly seen in diabetic patients.
2. CABG provides a more complete revascularisation in those with multivessel coronary artery disease.
3. CABG patients require less re-intervention.
4. CABG patients require less anti-anginal drugs.
5. PTCA is a less invasive procedure to the patient.
6. PTCA patients require a shorter initial hospital stay and so incur lower hospital costs but this is offset to some extent by repeat procedures.
7. PTCA patients return to work sooner than CABG patients but this difference disappears after a year of the procedure.

7. What can be done to maximise post-procedure benefit?

Measures which maximise benefit include:

1. Antiplatelet therapy – aspirin reduces saphenous vein graft closure[16]. This should be considered as standard care. In those patients with contraindications to aspirin, alternatives such as clopidogrel may be considered.
2. Pharmacological management of hyperlipidaemia – statin treatment in the post-bypass patient has been unequivocally demonstrated to retard progression of native coronary and vein graft disease[17]. Aggressive cholesterol reduction (target total cholesterol <4.8 mmol/l) also leads to a reduction in the requirement for repeat revascularisation (30% lower).
3. Cessation of smoking – there is strong evidence that this leads to less recurrent angina, improved function and fewer hospital admissions as well as improved survival[18]. Nicotine transdermal patches are effective in curtailing the addiction of smoking, as is the use of nicotine gum in addition to the patches.
4. Hormone replacement therapy – the American Heart Association and the American Fertility Society agree that hormone replacement therapy lowers mortality in women with moderate/severe coronary artery disease. In women post-CABG long-term survival is also improved with hormone replacement therapy[19].

8. Is there an age limit to CABG?

The elderly have a higher incidence of left main coronary artery disease, mutivessel disease, left ventricular impairment and reoperation, as well as other comorbid conditions. In the elderly, operative mortality has ranged from 5 to 20% for elective CABG. This is increased in emergency surgery[20].

However, despite the initial increased risk, functional recovery and sustained improvement in quality of life may be achieved in the majority of elderly patients. Age alone is not a contraindication and a decision with regard to proceeding to revascularisation should be made on an individual basis[6].

9. What are the future directions for revascularisation?

PTCA

As intracoronary stents have improved PTCA morbidity and mortality rates, attention is now being directed towards the reduction of in-stent restenosis. Techniques such as catheter-based gamma radiation, radioactive stents, gene therapy and local drug delivery systems are under evaluation[7]. As experience with stenting has increased, a number of studies have examined its use in more complex cases and in comparison with medical therapy, PTCA alone and CABG. The results of several such studies are awaited. There is evidence to suggest that in symptomatic patients with isolated proximal left anterior descending coronary stenosis, stenting is associated with a lower rate of restenosis and better clinical outcome than PTCA alone[24]. In the optimum PTCA compared with routine stent strategy trial (OPUS-1)[25], routine stent implantation was associated with better acute and long-term clinical outcomes with similar cost when compared with initial balloon angioplasty and provisional use of stents to treat suboptimal results. While most centres still consider left main stem stenosis an indication for CABG rather than PTCA and stenting, some studies have examined initial and long-term results of PTCA to the left main coronary artery and have suggested that this may be feasible in selected cases[26]. In a meta-analysis of randomised controlled trials of PTCA versus medical therapy for non-acute coronary heart disease, Butcher *et al.* concluded that PTCA may lead to a greater reduction in angina than medical treatment, but at the cost of more CABG[27]. These authors suggested that the available trials had not included enough patients to be able to draw firm conclusions regarding the effect of PTCA on myocardial infarction, death or subsequent revascularisation.

CABG

Techniques to minimise morbidity by less invasive methods for CABG and eliminating the use of cardiopulmonary bypass are already in the clinical arena. Minimally invasive CABG is performed through a left thoracotomy without cardiopulmonary bypass. This has reduced hospital stay and consequently hospital costs[21]. This procedure is still in its infancy.

Use of arterial conduits has made a major impact in long-term survival of CABG patients. Bilateral internal mammary artery grafting results in lower rates of recurrent angina and myocardial infarction[22]. Harvesting and use of the radial artery is also safe and reliable. Other arteries that can be considered as conduits include the right gastroepiploic artery and the inferior epigastric artery.

The importance of revascularisation, whether CABG or PTCA, upon prognosis and symptom control has been suggested in the recent prospective study of Hemingway *et al*[28].

10. Are there any alternatives to PTCA and CABG?

When conventional revascularisation techniques are unsuitable, transmyocardial revascularisation (TMR) or a similar catheter-based technique (Percutaneous transMyocardial Revascularisation, PMR,) may be considered an alternative in palliating symptoms. This procedure involves the use of a high-energy laser beam to create channels from the epicardial to the endocardial surface of the heart so allowing blood to perfuse ischaemic myocardium[23]. This mode of therapy is also in its infancy. Although early studies suggest encouraging results, full evaluation is required before it can be taken up on a wide scale. In the percutaneous transmyocardial laser revascularisation for severe angina (PACIFIC) randomised trial[29], percutaneous laser revascularisation was associated with increased exercise tolerance time, low morbidity, lower angina scores and increased quality of life. There was no effect upon survival.

References

1. Acierno LJ. Surgical modalities. In: *The History of Cardiology*. New York: The Parthenon Publishing Group, 1994:699–735.
2. Shiu MF. Interventional cardiac catheterisation: transluminal coronary angioplasty. In: Julian DG, Camm AJ, Fox KM, *et al.* (eds): *Diseases of the Heart*. Poole-Wilson PA: WB Saunders, 1996:1115–38.
3. Gray HH, on behalf of the council of the British cardiovascular intervention society. Cardiac interventional procedures in the UK 1992 to 1996. *Heart* 1999;**82 (Suppl. II)**:II10–17.
4. Belli G, Ellis SG, Topol EJ. Stenting for ischaemic heart disease. *Prog Cardiovasc Dis* 1997;**40**:159–82.
5. Gershlick AH, Baron J. Dealing with in-stent restenosis. *Heart* 1998;**79**:319–23.
6. Eagle KA, Guyton RA, Davidoff R, *et al.* ACC/AHA guidelines for coronary artery bypass graft surgery: a report of the American College of Cardiology/American Heart Association Task Force on Practice Guidelines (Committee to Revise the 1991 Guidelines for Coronary Artery Bypass Graft Surgery). *J Am Coll Cardiol* 1999;**34**:1262–346.
7. Gandhi MM, Dawkins KD. Intracoronary stents. *BMJ* 1999;**318**:650–53.
8. Serruys PW, Jaegere P, Kiemeneij F, *et al.* A comparison of balloon expandable stent implantation with balloon angioplasty in patients with coronary artery disease. *N Engl J Med* 1994;**331**:489–95.
9. Fischman DL, Leon MB, Baim DS, *et al.* A randomised comparison of coronary stent placement and balloon angioplasty in the treatment of coronary artery disease. *N Engl J Med* 1994;**331**:496–501.
10. O'Connor GT, Plume SK, Olmstead EM, *et al.* Multivariate prediction of in-hospital mortality associated with coronary artery bypass graft surgery: Northern New England Cardiovascular Disease Study Group. *Circulation* 1992;**85**:2110–18.
11. Grover FL, Johnson RR, Marshall G, *et al.* Factors predictive of operative mortality among coronary artery bypass subsets. *Ann Thorac Surg* 1993;**56**:1296–306.
12. Magovern JA, Sakert T, Magovern GJ, *et al.* A model that predicts morbidity and mortality after coronary artery bypass graft surgery. *J Am Coll Cardiol* 1996;**28**:1147–53.
13. Bypass Angioplasty Revascularisation Investigation (BARI) Investigators. Comparison of coronary artery bypass surgery with angioplasty in patients with multivessel disease. *N Engl J Med* 1996;**335**:217–25.
14. Chaitmen BR, Rosen AD, Williams DO, *et al.* Myocardial infarction and cardiac mortality in the Bypass Angioplasty Revascularisation Investigation (BARI) randomized trial. *Circulation* 1997;**96**:2162–70.
15. Goy JJ, Eeckhout E, Burnand B, *et al.* Coronary angioplasty versus left internal mammary artery grafting for isolated proximal left anterior descending artery stenosis. *Lancet* 1994;**343**:1449–53.
16. Sethi GK, Copeland JG, Goldman S, *et al.* Implications of preoperative administration of aspirin in patients undergoing coronary artery bypass grafting: Department of Veteran Affairs Cooperative Study on Antiplatelet Therapy. *J Am Coll Cardiol* 1990;**15**:15–20.
17. Post Coronary Artery Bypass Graft Trial Investigators. The effect of aggressive lowering of low-density lipoprotein cholesterol levels and low-dose anticoagulation on obstructive changes in saphenous-vein coronary-artery bypass grafts. *N Engl J Med* 1997;**336**:153–62.
18. Cavender JB, Rogers WJ, Fisher LD, *et al.* Effects of smoking on survival and morbidity in patients randomised to medical or surgical therapy in the Coronary Artery Surgery Study (CASS): 10-year follow-up: CASS Investigators. *J Am Coll Cardiol* 1992;**20**:287–94.
19. Sullivan JM, El-Zeky F, Vander Zwaag R, *et al.* Effect on survival of estrogen replacement therapy after coronary artery bypass grafting. *Am J Cardiol* 1997;**79**:847–50.
20. Hannan EL, Burke J. Effect of age on mortality in coronary artery bypass surgery in New York, 1991–1992. *Am Heart J* 1994;**128**:1184–91.
21. Borst C, Santamore WP, Smedira NG, *et al.* Minimally invasive coronary artery bypass grafting: on the beating heart and via limited access. *Ann Thorac Surg* 1997;**63**:S1–S5.
22. Cameron A, Davis KB, Green G, *et al.* Coronary bypass surgery with internal-thoracic-artery grafts – effects on survival over a 15-year period. *N Engl J Med* 1996;**334**:216–19.
23. Horvath KA, Cohn LH, Cooley DA, *et al.* Transmyocardial laser revascularisation: results of a multicenter trial with transmyocardial laser revascularisation used as sole therapy for end-stage coronary artery disease. *J Thorac Cardiovasc Surg* 1997;**113**:645–54.
24. Versaci F, Gaspardone A, Tomai F, *et al.* Comparison of coronary-artery stenting with angioplasty for isolated stenosis of the proximal left anterior descending coronary artery. *N Engl J Med* 1997;**336**:817–22.
25. Weaver WD, Reisman MA, Griffin JJ, *et al.* Optimum percutaneous transluminal coronary angioplasty compared with routine stent strategy trial (OPUS-1): a randomised trial. *Lancet* 2000;**355**:2199–203.
26. Kosuga K, Tamai H, Ueda K, *et al.* Initial and long-term results of angioplasty in unprotected left main coronary artery. *Am J Cardiol* 1999;**83**:32–37.
27. Butcher HC, Hengstler P, Schindler C, *et al.* Percutaneous transluminal coronary angioplasty versus medical treatment for non-acute coronary heart disease: meta-analysis of randomised controlled trials. *BMJ* 2000;**321**:73–7.
28. Hemingway H, Crook AM, Feder G, *et al.* Underuse of coronary revascularization procedures in patients considered appropriate candidates for revascularization. *N Eng J Med* 2001 (in press).
29. Oesterle SN, Sanborn TA, Ali N, *et al.* Percutaneous transmyocardial laser revascularisation for severe angina: the PACIFIC randomised trial. *Lancet* 2000;**356**:1705–10.

Index

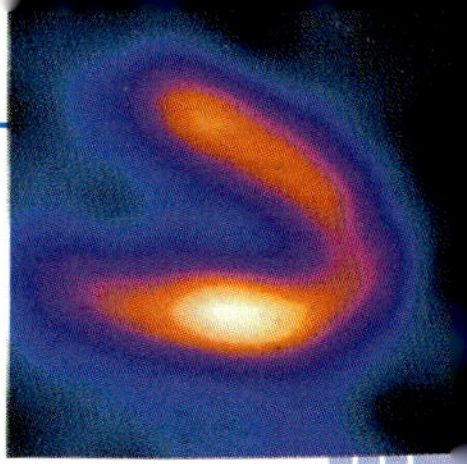

CHD – coronary heart disease/coronary artery disease
As the major subject of this book is 'Angina,' index entries have been kept to a minimum under this term and under 'Coronary artery disease.' Readers are advised to seek more specific entries.